D0109620

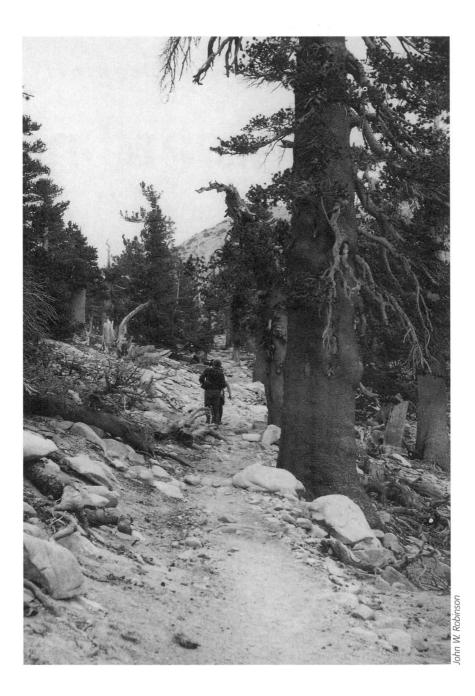

John W. Robinson

100 HIKES IN SOUTHERN CALIFORNIA

San Bernardino
MOUNTAIN
TRAILS

John W. Robinson
with David Money Harris

 WILDERNESS PRESS · BERKELEY, CA

San Bernardino Mountain Trails: 100 Hikes in Southern California

1st EDITION May 1972
2nd EDITION April 1975
3rd EDITION April 1979
4th EDITION August 1986
5th EDITION April 2003
6th EDITION January 2006

Copyright © 1972, 1975, 1979, 1986, 2003, 2006 by John W. Robinson
2004 update by Rick Whitaker
6th edition by David Money Harris

Front cover photo copyright © 2006 by David Muench
Interior photos, except where noted, by David Money Harris
Map design: Chris Salcedo/Blue Gecko, using data from John Robinson
          and David Money Harris, Laurence Jones, and U.S.G.S. topos
Cover design: Larry B. Van Dyke
Book design: Margaret Copeland/Terragraphics, and Larry B. Van Dyke
Book editor: Jessica Benner

ISBN-13 978-0-89997-409-5
ISBN-10 0-89997-409-0
UPC 7-19609-97409-3

Manufactured in the United States of America

Published by: **Wilderness Press**
               1200 5th Street
               Berkeley, CA 94710
               (800) 443-7227; FAX (510) 558-1696
               info@wildernesspress.com
               www.wildernesspress.com
Visit our website for a complete listing of our books and for ordering information.

Cover photos: The Pacific Crest Trail on San Gorgonio Mountain
Frontispiece: Lodgepole pines—high on the trail to San Gorgonio Mountain

All rights reserved. No part of this book may be reproduced in any form, or by any means electronic, mechanical, recording, or otherwise, without written permission from the publisher, except for brief quotations used in reviews.

SAFETY NOTICE: Although Wilderness Press and the author have made every attempt to ensure that the information in this book is accurate at press time, they are not responsible for any loss, damage, injury, or inconvenience that may occur to anyone while using this book. You are responsible for your own safety and health while in the wilderness. The fact that a trail is described in this book does not mean that it will be safe for you. Be aware that trail conditions can change from day to day. Always check local conditions and know your own limitations.

The San Bernardino Area

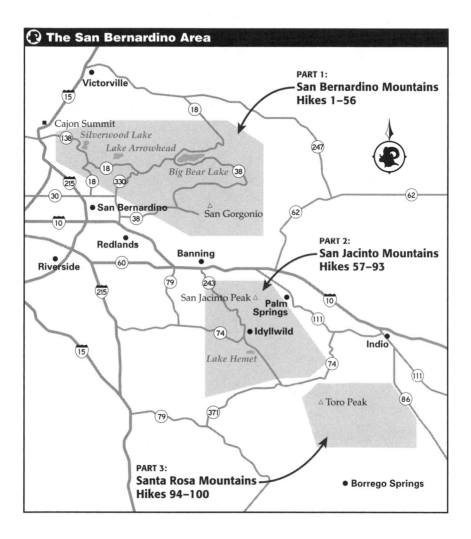

PART 1:
San Bernardino Mountains
Hikes 1–56

Victorville

Cajon Summit
Silverwood Lake
Lake Arrowhead
Big Bear Lake

San Bernardino
San Gorgonio

Redlands
Riverside
Banning

PART 2:
San Jacinto Mountains
Hikes 57–93

San Jacinto Peak △
Palm Springs
Idyllwild
Lake Hemet
Indio

△ Toro Peak

PART 3:
Santa Rosa Mountains
Hikes 94–100

● Borrego Springs

Contents

PART 1: The San Bernardino Mountains

PART 2: The San Jacinto Mountains

PART 3: The Santa Rosa Mountains

Prefaces to the 6th Edition

The San Bernardino and San Jacinto mountains have always held a special fascination for me. It's been more than half a century since I first ventured, on foot, from Poopout Hill to what we then called Slushy Meadows, up to Dollar Lake, and on to the gravely summit of San Gorgonio Mountain. Many times since, I have explored this wonderful high country, where stately lodgepole pine is the dominant conifer, snow patches linger into early summer, and the air is crisp with the chill of elevation. I have equally enjoyed the "sky island" of the high San Jacintos, its boulder-strewn ridges, and lush meadows. For more than five decades, I have walked the forest trails, forded the creeks, and scrambled up the peaks for far-reaching vistas.

In 1971, after completing *Trails of the Angeles*, a hiking guide to the San Gabriel Mountains, I suggested to Tom Winnett that Wilderness Press publish a trail guide to San Bernardino National Forest. Tom enthusiastically approved and a year later *San Bernardino Mountain Trails* appeared.

Over the next thirty-three years I rechecked the driving directions, rewalked the trails, reclimbed the peaks—all in an effort to keep the guidebook up to date. These were years of strenuous work. Unlike a novel, a trail guide is never finished; change is constant. Still, it was a labor of love, doing what I enjoy most, experiencing nature's beauty, meeting new friends.

Now, because of advancing age, the time has come to relinquish my work on *San Bernardino Mountain Trails*. My successor is a young energetic hiker who has already proved his worth by checking out many of the trail trips and making necessary revisions. David Money Harris is a Professor of Engineering at Harvey Mudd College in Claremont, who spends many of his non-teaching days rambling through the Southern California mountains.

I offer a heart-felt farewell to the many friends I have met, over all the years, on the trails. May you continue to enjoy walking the footpaths of the mountains we all love.

John W. Robinson
Fullerton, California
September 2005

It is an honor to be asked to update John Robinson's famous guidebook. My goal is to be faithful to the original flavor of the book while keeping it as accurate and current as possible.

I moved to Southern California from the Bay Area seven years ago and have been hiking the local mountains ever since. With each hike I take, Southern California feels more like home. Gazing up on a clear day at summits I have visited is like seeing old friends. While I had already hiked most of the major high points in the area, I had never even been aware of many of the more obscure hikes in this book. Checking them out has been a wonderful opportunity to make new acquaintances.

As John Robinson points out, change is constant. In this edition, I have eliminated ten trips, mostly because of access difficulties traversing private (or government and tribal) property. In their place, I have added ten new trips, with special emphasis on the Santa Rosa Mountains in the new National Monument and the increasingly popular Palm Springs area. Rick Whitaker scouted several of these new trips and flagged numerous corrections to other trips.

I have also endeavored to revise the driving directions. Navigating the maze of dirt roads to the trailhead may be the crux of many trips. I have provided trailhead GPS coordinates along with these new directions. Once on the trail, however, I leave you to navigate in the time-honored tradition with map, compass, and your own good sense.

I would like to thank the personnel of the Arrowhead, Sky Forest, Big Bear, Mill Creek, and Idyllwild ranger stations of San Bernardino National Forest and the Palm Springs field office of the Bureau of Land Management who offered invaluable advice about trail and campground changes and pointed out errors in the previous edition. Sharon Barsneck, Jim Foote, Melinda Lyon, Audrey Screnton, and Heidi Sellers were particularly generous with their time and knowledge.

Special thanks go to my friends who have hiked the trails with me, sharing splendid sunrises, glorious wildflowers, good conversation, spectacular vistas, and aching legs. Elizabeth Wenk and Janice Elliot helped identify plants and birds. I especially appreciate the company of the Uberjocks, Tony Condon and Joe Sheehy, during the many miles we have traveled together. And most of all, I thank my wife Jennifer for accompanying me on some trips and cheerfully sending me forth on others.

David Money Harris
Upland, California
October 2005

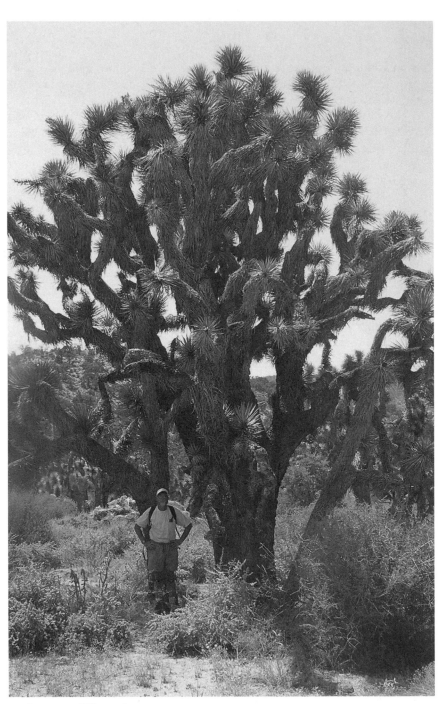

Joshua tree (Hike 27)

Introduction

San Bernardino National Forest sprawls over a generous portion of Southern California's mountain landscape. It begins atop Old Baldy in the San Gabriel Mountains and ends on the desert-tempered slopes of Toro Peak and Martinez Mountain in the Santa Rosa Mountains—100 miles in a great northwest-southeast arc. Within its bounds are all or part of four distinct mountain ranges—the eastern San Gabriels, the San Bernardinos, the San Jacintos, and the northern Santa Rosas (five ranges, if you consider Cahuilla Mountain to be separate from the San Jacintos).

Within the San Bernardino National Forest is all manner of mountain country. There are gentle flatlands and rolling hills, and there are sheer escarpments and rock-ribbed peaks that soar above everything else in Southern California. There are hot slopes smothered in thorny chaparral, and there are cool alpine forests of pine and fir. There are places where snow almost never falls, and there are spots where snowbanks linger half the year. There are sparkling mountain lakes and boggy meadows, quiet brooks and rushing streams. Often there are barrel cactuses and Joshua trees in close proximity to Jeffrey pines and incense-cedars. Perhaps no other national forest in the United States contains such variety.

Humans have made an indelible mark on much of this landscape. We have built a maze of roads, and have erected a multitude of homes, resorts, and places of business high up in the forest country. Some areas—Crestline, Lake Arrowhead, Big Bear, Idyllwild—are so urbanized that they differ little from the cities below. About 44,000 people make their permanent home in the San Bernardino Mountains.

Yet there is wilderness here in these overused mountains, places where civilization—either by nature's design or human foresight—has left the mountains to themselves. Here, deep in the forest, alongside an alder-canopied stream or high on a rocky crag, you can relax and contemplate and enjoy nature's solitude. You can breathe the restoring scents of forest and chaparral, and listen to the quiet sounds of the earth. You can come to understand the true value of wilderness to a civilization that too often places artificial values before real ones.

1

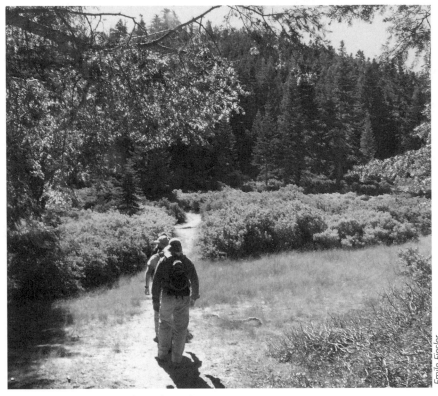

Entering the Berry Patch (Hike 58)

The largest wilderness regions in San Bernardino National Forest are the wild areas around San Gorgonio Mountain and San Jacinto Peak, set aside to remain forever in their natural, pristine state. Here is the highest mountain country in Southern California and, in the eyes of many, the most delightful. Besides these two official wild areas, there are many other parts of the mountains where, by reason of remoteness or difficulty of access, human touch has been minimal. These are scattered throughout the mountains, some of them quite close to overused areas—the Pinnacles country north of Lake Arrowhead, lower Holcomb and Deep creeks, the bouldered slopes above Big Bear Lake, the Heart Bar country, Yucaipa Ridge, the palm-and-pinyon country on the desert slopes of the San Jacintos, the lonely Santa Rosas, to name the best.

This guidebook attempts to acquaint Southern Californians—and others—with the intimate parts of San Bernardino National Forest, the regions away from the highway where nature still reigns relatively undisturbed. The 100 hiking trips in this book take the reader and prospective hiker into almost every nook and cranny of the mountains. They vary from easy one-hour strolls to all-day and overnight rambles involving many miles of walking and much elevation change—excursions to satisfy the novice and challenge the veteran.

There is one overriding requirement—you must like to walk and be willing to forgo the comforts of civilization for periods ranging from a few short hours to several days.

Trails and fire roads crisscross much of San Bernardino National Forest, some well maintained and easy to follow, others almost-forgotten byways of the past, eroded and overgrown in spots. The great majority of trips in this guidebook are on maintained trails, and these should present no problems to the hiker. However, I have included a handful of cross-country scrambles and trailless peak climbs in areas well worth visiting but not served by standard routes. For these trips, directions have been presented in greater detail.

More so than any other national forest in California, and perhaps in the entire nation, San Bernardino National Forest is dotted with private holdings. This is particularly so in the urban belt of the San Bernardino Mountains that extends from Crestline eastward through Twin Peaks, Blue Jay, Lake Arrowhead, Running Springs, Green Valley, to Big Bear; and in the Idyllwild area of the San Jacinto Mountains. Besides these extensive developed areas, there are literally hundreds of private holdings ranging in size from fifty or more acres down to an acre or less. Only the San Gorgonio Wilderness, San Jacinto State Park, the San Jacinto Wilderness, the Santa Rosa Wilderness, and the newly established San Jacinto and Santa Rosa Mountains National Monument are relatively inviolate. Several of the trail trips described in this guidebook pass through or alongside private property. The hiker attempting these trips may be confronted with a locked gate or an irate property owner. Trips that pass through non-public land are so indicated in the trip description. To avoid disappointment, contact the nearest ranger district to learn the latest information on accessibility.

I have walked, recorded, and researched all the trips in this guide. Every effort has been made to present the information as accurately and as explicitly as possible. Nevertheless, the prospective hiker should be aware that several factors—the rapid growth of chaparral, fire, flood, and the continual reworking of trails—may make some of this information out-of-date in a short time. Such changes will probably affect only a few of the trips described here, but if you are unfamiliar with the area in which you plan to hike, it is best to inquire at a ranger station before your trip.

The trail trips have been graded, based on my evaluation, as "easy," "moderate," "strenuous," or "very strenuous." An "easy" trip is usually four miles or less in horizontal distance, with less than 500' elevation gain—suitable for beginners and children. A "moderate" trip—including the majority here—is a five-to-ten-mile hike, usually with less than 2500' elevation difference. You should be in fair physical condition for these, and children under 12 might find the going difficult. "Strenuous" trips are all-day rambles involving many miles of hiking and much elevation gain and loss; they are only for those in top physical condition and with hiking experience. "Very strenuous" trips involve at least a vertical mile of elevation gain and include some of the classic physical challenges of Southern California. The most important criteria for grading a trip are mileage covered, elevation gain and loss, and condition of the trail. Of less significance are accessibility of terrain, availability of water, exposure to sun, and ground cover. Obviously, some of the latter criteria depend on the weather and time of year: a 3-mile hike over open chaparral slopes can be miserable under the hot August sun but delightful in January's cool breeze and cloudiness.

A season recommendation is included for each trip. This classification is particularly important in the lower, south- and west-facing parts of the mountains; due to fire danger these sections may be closed until the first appreciable rain.

This book is entitled *San Bernardino Mountain Trails* because the mountain regions covered are predominantly in San Bernardino National Forest. There are two exceptions. The western end of San Bernardino National Forest extends into the San Gabriel Mountains and this section is included in the companion volume *Trails of the Angeles*. To make up for this absence, the entire Santa Rosa Range is covered in this guide, even though San Bernardino National Forest encompasses only the northern half. So, the reader comes out even.

It is my earnest desire that this guidebook will provide the prospective mountain visitor with the knowledge that can make an outing in the San Bernardinos, San Jacintos, or Santa Rosas an enjoyable and meaningful experience. If you learn and heed forest regulations, follow route directions, become familiar with the area, have proper equipment, and use good sense, you will thoroughly appreciate your intimacy with the mountains. Never leave the trailhead without this preparation. The mountains are no place to travel alone, unbriefed, ill-equipped, or in poor condition. Enter their portals with the enthusiasm of adventure tempered with respect, forethought, and common sense. The mountains belong to those who are wise as well as willing.

Hiking Hints

Some hikers have emerged from the mountains with the scent of laurel and pine on their clothing and with dust on their boots, tired but enriched—both physically and mentally—by their wilderness experience. Others have stumbled out of the mountains exhausted, footsore, sunburned, dehydrated, chilled, with clothing and skin torn by thorny chaparral, or soaked to the bone by unexpected downpour, sadder but wiser for their ordeal. Some have had to be carried out. And a few have not come out.

An outing in the mountains can be many things—fabulous, pleasant, unpleasant, harrowing, or disastrous. How it turns out depends to a large degree on you—your preparation, your clothing and equipment, your physical condition, and your good sense.

Following are some hints to make your mountain trip an enjoyable and rewarding experience.

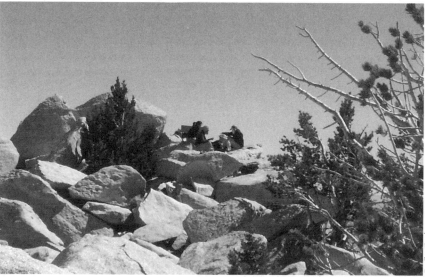

Summit team, San Jacinto Peak

Emile Fiesler

Preparation

Choose a trip that suits your ability. If you have never hiked before, visit Little Bear Creek or Long Valley—something in the "easy" category. As you gain experience and learn the feel of mountain travel, graduate to something in the "moderate" class. Do not undertake a "strenuous" outing until you are both experienced and in top physical condition.

Become familiar with the terrain and landscape features of the area you plan to visit by studying a good map beforehand. It may be advisable to check with the Forest Service before your trip, particularly if you plan to walk a trail not regularly maintained (such trails are so indicated in this guide). Most rangers on duty at the National Forest ranger stations are only too glad to help, and few people know the mountains better than they. Or contact San Bernardino National Forest headquarters at 1824 South Commercenter Circle, San Bernardino, CA 92408. Phone: (909) 382-2600.

The San Gorgonio Wilderness Association posts snow and camping conditions for the wilderness area at: www.sgwa.org/trails.htm.

Permits

If you plan to visit the San Gorgonio Wilderness, the San Jacinto Wilderness or Mount San Jacinto State Wilderness, you must obtain a wilderness permit first. The permit is free to anyone who will agree to follow some simple rules intended to protect the visitor as well as the wilderness. Groups are limited to 12 people.

To obtain the permit, visit or write to one of the ranger stations listed in Appendix 1. There are quotas on permits for some of the most popular trails and these quotas are often filled well in advance on summer weekends. For hikes in the San Jacinto Wilderness, a single wilderness permit from either the Forest Service or State Park is sufficient for hikes spanning the two agencies.

If you plan to camp overnight in the San Bernardino National Forest, you are required to obtain a campfire permit, available from most ranger stations.

A Forest Adventure Pass is required for all vehicles parking in any of the four national forests of Southern California—San Bernardino, Cleveland, Angeles, Los Padres. A one-day pass is $5; an annual pass is $30; for senior citizens, it is $15. The pass can be purchased at Forest Service stations and some mountain stores. The Golden Eagle Pass ($65) may be a better deal because it also covers all National Parks and many other federal lands.

The Forest Adventure Pass is part of the 2005 Recreation Enhancement Act (formerly the 1996 Recreation Fee Demonstration Program) to collect user fees because the Forest Service receives inadequate federal funding. Nevertheless, it seems odd that the Forest Service should subsidize construction of backcountry roads for timber and mining interests, then charge hikers to park on these same roads. This author (Harris) and many others believe that the Forest Service should receive proper funding from our tax dollars and from commercial users, not from parking fees on public lands.

Purchasing a day pass is a logistical problem for long day hikes that start before the stores open. At the time of this writing, if you receive a ticket for not displaying a pass, you can resolve it by purchasing and sending in a day pass. Hence, it may be more practical to purchase the day pass after the hike than before.

Access to trailheads

Finding and reaching the trailhead may be half the challenge for many of these trips. The author has spent hours searching for dirt roads that are easy to miss from the highway. Fortunately, highways have mileage marker signs. For example 038 SBD 53.50 is a marker at mile 53.50 on Highway 38 in San Bernardino County. Directions are often given relative to these markers.

The San Bernardino National Forest map, published by the Forest Service and available at most ranger stations, provides a reasonably up-to-date rendition of the dirt roads and trailheads in both the San Bernardino and San Jacinto mountains. AAA publishes a San Bernardino Mountains Guide Map that is also helpful, though less complete.

A Global Positioning Satellite (**GPS**) receiver also can be helpful to locate trailheads. Where possible, this edition provides GPS coordinates for the start of a hike. Automotive GPS units with a good database of dirt roads (such as that provided with Garmin units) can provide driving directions from your house all the way to the trailhead. Appendix 3 provides GPS waypoints for most trailheads.

The condition of dirt roads changes rapidly. At the time of this writing, nearly all trailheads can be reached with an ordinary passenger car so long as it is driven carefully. On dirt roads listed as "fair" or "poor," a high clearance 4WD vehicle is more likely to arrive unscathed. Exercise good judgment.

Clothing

Mountain weather can vary considerably, even within a few hours. It is best to come prepared for both warm and cool temperatures with several layers of clothing—shirt, sweater and windbreaker, for example—that can be put on or peeled off as needed. This is particularly advisable if you plan to climb any of the high peaks.

Short pants may be satisfactory when walking a fire road or rambling through an open forest at middle elevations, but they are miserable for thrashing through chaparral. If any part of your trip is through this elfin forest, wear sturdy long pants—and expect to get them torn.

Choice of headgear depends on the hiker. If you sunburn easily, you will probably want a hat with generous brim. If the weather looks threatening, bring raingear.

Modern medical knowledge has linked skin damage and skin cancer with long periods of skin exposure to the sun. Long pants, a good hat, and generous sunscreen are recommended.

Footgear

If the walk is short and on good trail, tennis shoes are adequate. But if the trip is long or over rough terrain, a pair of sturdy boots, preferably with deep tread, should be worn.

Properly fitting shoes and close-fitting, heavy-duty socks are essential to prevent blisters and sore feet. A mistake in footwear can ruin your trip. Break in new boots on short walks before you attempt a long hike. If you blister easily, carry moleskin, and use it at the first hint of oncoming trouble.

Equipment

A day hike in the mountains requires little in the way of equipment. It is surprising how many novices overburden themselves with large packs, extra clothing, too much or too heavy food, hunting knives, and miscellaneous gadgets.

Still, there are essentials that all hikers should carry. These include a full water bottle, a first-aid kit, an area map, and some food. If you are doing any cross-country hiking, a compass is advisable and a topographic map is virtually a requirement. You will probably want to bring a camera. To carry all this, a lightweight daypack is advisable, preferably with a waistband to better distribute the weight.

An overnight outing, of course, requires more (see *Backpacking* below).

Food

Trail menus vary considerably, and there is little agreement among experts about what foods are best. Sandwiches, cheese, fruit, nuts, cookies, and candy are probably the most popular trail foods. A planned, balanced diet is necessary only on an outing of several days.

What you eat is not nearly so important as how much you eat, and when. Small lunches plus snacks along the trail are best, because exertion after a feast causes competition for blood between stomach and hiking muscles, and leads to indigestion and weakness.

As important as food on a hike is liquid. Without enough water, exertion and heat dehydrate the body surprisingly soon and cause marked muscular weakness. Unless you are walking alongside a stream, bring a full water bottle—several if the weather is hot and your walk is long.

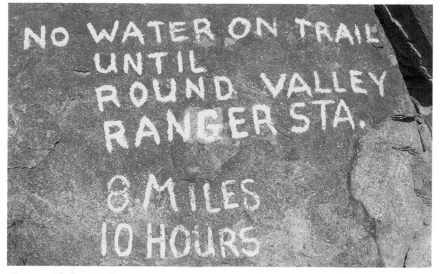

Sign on Skyline Trail

Giardia has made its appearance here. All water should be boiled, treated or filtered first.

On the trail

Walking a mountain trail is not as simple as one might think. An enjoyable hike requires proper pace and rest stops, knowledge of the terrain, correct reading of trail signs and, above all, good judgment.

Unless you are training for the Olympics, a trail hike should not be a race to your destination and back. Start out slowly, easing your muscles into condition. Work up to the steady, rhythmic pace that suits you best. Your best trail speed is one at which you are working but not panting, and you feel you can continue almost indefinitely. When the trail steepens, shorten your steps but maintain your rhythm. Take short rests at moderate intervals, rather than stopping too frequently or for too long a time. If you are exceeding your ability, symptoms of exhaustion soon set in: sore or cramped leg muscles, profuse sweating, pounding pulse, headache, dizziness, redness of the face. Not only do these lessen your enjoyment, but a tired hiker is more accident-prone. The speedster who rushes up the trail, then collapses in a panting heap, is usually overtaken before long by the leisurely hiker. "Who goes into the mountains fast, comes out last," says an old proverb.

Stay on the trail. Short cuts not only break down the trail (see *Mountain Courtesy* below) but can lead you astray. Probably the greatest temptation is to cut switchbacks—but sometimes the last zigzag doesn't zag, and you find yourself stumbling down a steep talus slope to nowhere, or thrashing through thorny brush in the wrong direction. When you finally realize your mistake, you are faced with the unpleasant necessity of churning back up the loose talus or beating through an ocean of chaparral—a painful, time-consuming object lesson in mountain sense.

When you come to a marked trail junction, read the sign carefully. If a junction is unmarked, consult your map and observe the surrounding land-marks to keep yourself oriented. If the trail seems to disappear in brush or boulders, look ahead for the way you think it should go; most trails take the obvious route. Look for *ducks* (several stones piled atop one another) that indicate the route. If you still can't find the trail, and you are not experienced in cross-country travel, it is better to return the way you came rather than risk getting lost.

Off the trail

Although trails crisscross San Bernardino National Forest, there are some places they don't go—the length of Deep Creek in the San Bernardinos, and up Cornell Peak in the San Jacintos, for example. To reach these objectives, you must leave the established footpath and travel cross-country. Off-trail hiking, except for very short distances, is not for beginners. Attempt it only if you are an experienced hiker, and then never alone.

Cross-country hiking in the San Bernardinos and San Jacintos is practical only in parts of the mountains—at higher elevations, along ridgetops and along streambeds. In lower-elevation chaparral it is virtually impossible.

If you are planning a trip that is part cross-country, be sure you know the terrain, the landmarks, the ground cover and the distance. Obtain a topo-graphic map of the area and plan your route beforehand. Before you leave road or trail, make a visual survey of the region, noting the locations of land-marks. Continue this careful observation as you hike; look back at land-marks you'll want to use on the return trip—it's surprising how different the country sometimes looks when you're going the other way.

Without question, the most unpleasant type of cross-country travel is bushwhacking—an ordeal you should avoid whenever possible. One mile through unyielding chaparral is as difficult and tiring as 6 or 8 miles on trail, and much rougher on your clothing. If you must bush-whack, seek out ter-rain where the elfin forest is less dense—along ridges, in gullies, over recent-ly burned areas. Chaparral also is thinner on shady, north-facing slopes than on sun-drenched, south-facing slopes. When entering a brushy area, secure loose items of clothing and equipment. It's mighty tough to retrace your exact route to find a lost camera or canteen.

On slopes of loose talus or scree, tread lightly; even the most careful walk-er cannot avoid dislodging a few rocks or triggering a slide. Solid-looking boulders may be precariously balanced; you must be ever-ready to leap nim-bly aside when a foothold gives way.

Stream crossing is an art thoroughly mastered by few, and few hikers have never dampened their boots. If you cannot find a dry crossing—a series of stepping-stones or a strategically located log—you must wade. It is better to wade the widest part of the stream, where the water is shallower and the current is slower. If the streambed rocks are smooth, wade across barefoot. If they are sharp-edged, remove your socks and wear your boots across. Then drain your boots, dry your feet, and replace socks and boots.

Hiking over snow can be a pleasure if the grade is gentle and the snow firm but not icy. It can be tedious if the sun has softened the snow so much that you break through at every step. And it can be extremely dangerous if the slope is steep and the snow icy, as it often is in higher elevations during late winter and spring. If you plan to snow-hike, a pair of boots with deep tread are a necessity, preferably treated with a waterproof wax and worn with gaiters (waterproof leggings covering the upper part of the boot and part of the pant leg) to keep your feet dry. An ice axe, and knowledge of how to use it, is a requirement for steep snow slopes. Serious climbing on snow and ice, requiring ice axe, crampons, and rope, is only for skilled mountaineers. If you are interested, the Sierra Club offers a mountaineering course.

Rock climbing

Rock climbers have graded mountain routes into five categories, ranging from Class 1 (hiking) to Class 5 (climbing a vertical or overhanging cliff). You won't find much above Class 1 or 2 in these mountains, but there are some peaks whose ascent by certain routes involves some steep rock-scrambling—categorized as Class 3. The Pinnacles and Cornell Peak are examples. Class 3 climbing requires great caution. Move slowly, and test every handhold and foothold before shifting your weight. Take extra care on the descent, for this is when most accidents occur. Wear boots with deep tread for traction on rock. Tahquitz Rock above Idyllwild is a favorite practice area for advanced rock climbers.

Backpacking

San Bernardino National Forest offers superb opportunities for overnight backpack trips—particularly in the San Gorgonio and San Jacinto wilderness areas. The Forest Service maintains a number of overnight trail camps in these and other areas, many of them in delightful sylvan haunts away from the markings of civilization.

Most important is your choice of a pack itself. A wrong choice can cause an aching back and make backpacking a disagreeable experience. There are two main types of packs—internal frame and external frame packs—and each has its advantages. While both types of pack place most of the weight on your hips rather than on your shoulders, internal frame packs are superior for hiking over uneven terrain because they keep the load close to your body, allow for more upper-body motion, and have a lower center of gravity than external frame packs. They also can carry a heavier load. External frame packs hold the weight away from your back, making them cooler in warm weather. They provide more outside pockets and easier access to their contents, and are also less expensive than their internal frame counterparts.

For a good night's rest, you need a good sleeping bag. Down is the most efficient material for keeping you warm. Synthetic bags provide less warmth per unit of weight than down bags, making them heavier and bulkier. The advantages of synthetic bags are that they cost less, dry more quickly, and retain some insulating value when wet. For summertime trips in elevations below 8000 feet, chances are that nights in these mountains will be mild, and a cheaper bag will be adequate. If you're a winter or spring backpacker, or if you plan to camp at any of the high trail camps in the two wild areas, better go with a down bag. "Mummy" and rectangular shaped bags each have their adherents. Some people cannot tolerate the close fit of the mummy style, despite its superior thermal and weight characteristics.

Other backpacking essentials include warm clothing, raingear, plastic ground cloth, air mattress or foam pad, utensils, cooking gear, flashlight, first-aid kit, snakebite kit, matches, and toilet paper. During rainy season (winter and spring) tote a waterproof tent or—much less expensive—a plastic "tube tent" held up by nylon line.

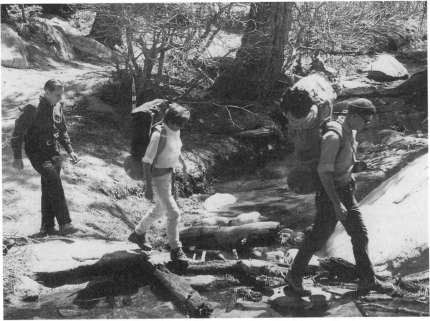

John W. Robinson

Backpackers crossing Willow Creek in San Jacinto Wilderness

Camping

You are required to obtain a campfire permit, obtainable at most ranger stations, if you plan to camp overnight in San Bernardino National Forest. If your trip is in the San Gorgonio Wilderness (federal), the San Jacinto Wilderness (federal), or the San Jacinto State Wilderness, you must obtain a wilderness permit (which includes permission for a campfire where applicable). Camp only in established trail camps and build your fire only in campground stoves or fire rings; *open fires are not allowed.* Certain parts of the National Forest ban campfires entirely, especially during periods of high fire danger. In the San Jacinto Wilderness (federal) the Forest Service has delineated camping zones; yellow posts to indicate camping areas within each zone. At present, you do not need to obtain a wilderness permit to enter the new Santa Rosa Wilderness.

Portions of the National Forest have been ravaged by bark beetles, leaving stands of dead trees waiting to topple. It is prudent to camp and picnic away from these trees.

Emergencies

The Sierra Madre Search and Rescue Team, without doubt the top mountain-rescue organization in Southern California, says that in the great majority of mountain emergencies in which a hiker is lost or injured, he or she 1) set off alone, 2) did not leave an itinerary or a planned return time, and/or 3) took a "short cut" off the established trail. If you do all three, and are a relatively inexperienced mountaineer, you are inviting trouble. However, even the experienced and careful hiker may have a crisis. Knowing what to do in an emergency may save your life.

The first rule for survival in any outdoor emergency—be it losing your way, injury, snakebite, storm or fire—is common sense: make a calm, reasoned judgment of the situation and act accordingly. The biggest threat to survival is panic. Panicky hikers have been known to throw away their supplies and wander aimlessly for miles. According to mountain-rescue experts, 8 of 10 survival-situation fatalities could have been prevented if the hiker had known survival techniques and had used common sense.

Getting lost is by far the most common crisis faced by hikers. If you ever face this prospect, awareness of several basic rules should spare you unnecessary strain, fatigue, or injury, and maybe even your life. The minute you realize you are lost, stop and appraise the situation. If you are reasonably certain of your general location and have map and compass, try to retrace your steps, looking always for footprints and familiar landmarks. You may want to climb a nearby high point to survey the terrain for landmarks. Never take what you think is a "short cut" over unfamiliar terrain; you stand a chance of becoming hopelessly tangled in thorny chaparral or slipping down a steep slope. If you are uncertain of your whereabouts, stay put. Never try to find your way at night.

If you've told people where you were going (and never enter the mountains on foot without telling someone your planned itinerary), a search will be made, probably the next day. Try to stay warm by huddling against a tree or by using branches, bark or pine needles to build a primitive shelter. Don't search extensively for food; water is far more critical. To attract help from the air (search-and-rescue teams make much use of the helicopter nowadays) hang out bright-colored clothing or other objects, but do not under any circumstances start a fire—you could burn down the forest, endangering your life and the lives of many others. A common distress signal is three signs, visible or audible, repeated at intervals—for example, three bright objects placed in a row or three shouts. If you manage to find your way out on your own, immediately notify the Forest Service or Sheriff's Office so that the search can be ended.

The best way to avoid being trapped in a storm is to stay out of the mountains when the weather is threatening. If you are caught in a sudden blizzard at higher elevations, descend as rapidly as you can with safety, but don't start down unfamiliar slopes that might lead to dropoffs or to box canyons. Stay off ridges and open saddles, where wind velocity often becomes extreme. At lower elevations, your worry is water rather than snow or wind. Stay clear of canyon bottoms and gullies that are vulnerable to flash floods. If you're on the trail, stay on it. If you try a short cut, your anxiety to get out, combined with the decreased visibility, could get you hopelessly lost. If you can't make it out, seek shelter in the hollow of a tree or under a rock overhang, away from the raging stream.

Fire in the Southern California mountains can be a fearful thing. Chaparral, especially when it's tinder-dry in late summer and fall, burns with unbelievable intensity, and wind can cause a brush fire to rampage at enormous speeds. If you see a fire in the mountains, even one that seems a safe distance away, get out fast and notify the Forest Service—the fire could be upon you before you realize it. If you are confronted by a close-at-hand brush fire, you must act fast. Determine the wind direction—fire moves much more rapidly downwind—and move laterally from that direction. Seek slopes and gullies where chaparral is sparse or absent—the fire may pass around these pockets. Or seek the refuge of a stream, preferably where brush does not crowd the banks. About 90% of Southern California forest and brush fires are caused by human carelessness, so make certain that no one in your party contributes to this tragic destruction.

Mountain Courtesy

Traveling a mountain trail, away from centers of civilization, is a unique experience in Southern California living. It brings intimate association with nature—communion with the earth, the forest, the chaparral, the wildlife, the clear sky. A great responsibility accompanies this experience—the obligation to keep the mountains as you find them. Being considerate of the wilderness rights of others will make the mountain adventures of those who follow equally rewarding.

As a mountain visitor, you should become familiar with the rules of wilderness courtesy outlined below.

Trails

Cutting switchbacks breaks down trails and hastens erosion. Take care not to dislodge rocks that might fall on hikers below you. Improve and preserve trails, as by clearing away loose rocks (carefully) and removing branches. Report any trail damage and broken or misplaced signs to a ranger.

Off Trail

Restrain the impulse to blaze trees or to build ducks where it's not essential. Let other hikers find their own way as you did.

Campgrounds

Spread your gear in an already-cleared area, and build your fire in a campground stove. Don't disarrange the camp by making hard-to-eradicate ramparts of rock for fireplaces or windbreaks. Rig tents and tarps with line tied to rocks or trees; never put nails in trees. For your campfire, use fallen wood or carry your own wood in rather than cutting standing trees or breaking off branches. Use the campground latrine. Place litter in the litter can or carry it out. Leave your campsite cleaner than you found it. Camp 200 feet or more from creeks and lakes.

Fire

Fire is the greatest danger in the Southern California mountains; act accordingly. Smoke only in cleared areas along the trail. Report a mountain fire immediately to the Forest Service. Campfires are not permitted in many portions of the San Bernardino National Forest, especially during times of high fire hazard in the summer and fall. Check regulations with the ranger station before planning to have a campfire.

Litter

Along the trail, place candy wrappers, raisin boxes, orange peels, etc. in your pocket or pack for later disposal; throw nothing on the trail. Pick up litter you find along the trail or in camp. More than almost anything else, litter detracts from the wilderness scene. Remember, you can take it with you.

Noise

Boisterous conduct is out of harmony in a wilderness experience. Be a considerate hiker and camper. Don't ruin another's enjoyment of the mountains.

Good Samaritanship

Human life and well-being take precedence over everything else—in the mountains as elsewhere. If a hiker or camper is in trouble, help in any way you can. Indifference is a moral crime. Give comfort or first aid; then hurry to a ranger station for help.

Maps

When you are hiking, it is important to know where you are in relation to roads, campgrounds, landmarks, etc. and to know the lay of the land in general. For learning these things there is no substitute for a good map. Unless your trip is very short, and over a well-marked route, you should carry a map.

There are several types of maps readily available that will give you the picture you need of San Bernardino National Forest and its adjacent mountain areas. Each type has its advantages and its disadvantages.

1. The large custom-designed fold-out map at the back of this book shows all the hikes in this book, including trailheads, access roads, and overlaps with forest service roads and other trails, such as the Pacific Crest Trail. You'll also find points-of-interest mentioned in the text, watercourses, ranger stations, picnic and camping areas, and other information you might not find anywhere else. This map will help you locate trails and get the big picture. However, the topographic maps listed below provide substantially more detail that is essential if you plan to hike off trail.

2. Tom Harrison Maps produces topographic maps for the San Gorgonio Wilderness and San Jacinto Wilderness. These maps are laminated and show trail mileage. They can be purchased at most outdoor stores or from www.tomharrisonmaps.com for $8.95. They are more convenient and withstand abuse better than the U.S. Forest Service wilderness maps.

3. The U.S. Forest Service provides topographic maps of the San Gorgonio, San Jacinto, and Santa Rosa wildernesses are available for $6.00–$8.00. These maps can be obtained at most ranger stations, at outdoor stores, or at www.fs.fed.us/recreation/nationalforeststore/nfs_order_form.html

4. Earthwalk Press publishes a laminated topographic map titled Anza-Borrego Desert Region Recreation Map that covers the southern Santa Rosa region as well as the Anza-Borrego Desert. It is sold in local hiking stores or can be ordered from stores such as The Globe Corner Bookstore (www.globecorner.com) for $7.95.

5. The US Geological Survey (USGS) 7.5′ series of topographic maps cover the entire region; each map covers about 7 x 9 miles and has 40-foot contour intervals. They provide excellent detail, but cover such a small area that 29 separate maps are necessary to cover all the hikes in this book. These maps are sold at some outdoor shops or at store.usgs.gov for $6.00.

◑ Index to 7.5′ USGS topographic maps

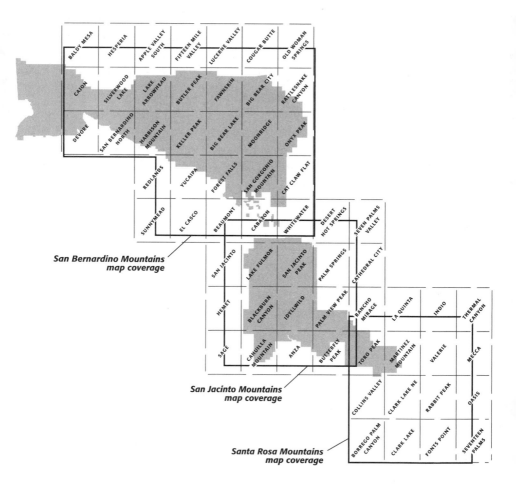

San Bernardino Mountains map coverage

San Jacinto Mountains map coverage

Santa Rosa Mountains map coverage

One Hundred Hikes

How this Book is Organized

The hiking trips in this guide are arranged by geographical area, generally northwest to southeast, from Cajon Pass at the west end of the San Bernardinos to Rabbit Peak at the southern end of the Santa Rosas. The first section covers the San Bernardino Mountains, with the largest concentration of hikes in the San Gorgonio Wilderness. The next section covers the San Jacinto Mountains, concentrated in Mount San Jacinto State Park and the San Jacinto Wilderness, along with a cluster in Palm Canyon. The final section covers the rugged Santa Rosa Mountains.

The guide is divided into three parts—The San Bernardino Mountains, the San Jacinto Mountains and the Santa Rosa Mountains—with introductory information on each mountain range preceding the trips for that range.

Information about each trip is divided into three parts:

The **Hike** section gives vital statistics: where the hike starts and ends; the walking mileage and elevation gain or loss; a rating of easy, moderate, strenuous, or very strenuous; the best time of year to make the trip; and the appropriate topographic map or maps.

The **Features** section tells something of what you will see on the trip, and gives information on the natural and human history of the area. It also contains suggestions for the particular trip, such as, wear deep-tread boots, or bring fishing rod.

The **Description** section details the driving and hiking route. The driving directions are kept to the necessary minimum, but the walking route is described in detail. Also, the hiking-route options that a trip offers are presented.

If you are a dedicated hiker who enjoys exploring the Southern California mountains on foot, the trips listed here are just a beginning. Many more than 100 hikes are possible, crisscrossed as these mountains are by roads, trails and cross-country routes. Furthermore, various combinations of routes described here are possible, particularly if you can arrange car shuttles. You could spend a decade rambling through these mountains and still not fully know them.

Summary of Hikes

The tables below sort the hikes by best season and by length. The season is classified as *warm*, *cool*, or *any*. Warm season hikes in the high mountains are usually covered by snow in the winter. Cool season hikes in the deserts can be dangerously hot in the summer. Many strenuous day trips can be done as a moderate backpack.

Any Season

	Hike	Distance (in miles)	Elevation Gain (in feet)
3	Heart Rock	2	300
6	Deep Creek Hot Springs	3	700
13	Upper Deep Creek	4	500
26	Silver Peak	4	1000
9	Little Bear Creek	5	800
10	Deep Creek	5	500
81	Cedar Spring	5.5	1700
5	Arrowhead Peak	6	1400
57	Black Mountain	7	2600
80	Palm View Peak	7	2200
39	Siberia Creek Trail Camp from Seven Pines	8	600
21	Siberia Creek Trail Camp from Snow Valley	8.5	2000
18	Cox Creek	9	600
79	Apache Peak	12	2600
82	Thomas Mountain	12	2100
78	Antsell Rock	16	2700

Warm Season

	Hike	Distance (in miles)	Elevation Gain (in feet)
12	Heaps Peak Arboretum	0.7	100
29	Champion Lodgepole Pine	1	50
38	Ponderosa Nature Trail	1	150
53	Big Falls	1	200
60	North Fork, San Jacinto River	1 to 4	200
28	Castle Rock	2	700
74	Lily Rock	2	1500
76	Ernie Maxwell Scenic Trail	2.5	300
20	Little Green Valley	3	700
14	Holcomb Crossing Trail Camp	6	900
25	Gold Mountain	4	1000

Hike	Distance (in miles)	Elevation Gain (in feet)
19 Exploration Trail	4	1300
36 Fish Creek Meadow	5	650
84 Long, Round, and Tamarack Valleys	5	600
23 Delamar Mountain	5	1000
46 Johns Meadow	5.5	600
22 Grays Peak	6	1200
31 Grand View Point	6	1200
67 Skunk Cabbage Meadow	6	1600
51 Alger Creek Trail Camp	6.5	1400
24 Bertha Peak	7	1400
33 Sugarloaf Mountain from Wildhorse Meadows	7	1300
64 Suicide Rock	7	1900
71 Tahquitz Valley	7	1700
77 Tahquitz Peak via South Ridge Trail	7	2300
61 Deer Springs	7.5	2600
34 Wildhorse Creek	8	1400
94 Alta Seca Bench	8	800
73 Tahquitz Peak via Saddle Junction	8.5	2400
35 Santa Ana River Headwaters	9	800
40 South Fork Meadows	9	1600
55 Galena Peak	9	3200
32 Sugarloaf Mountain from Green Canyon	10	2000
37 Fish Creek	11	1900
65 Strawberry–Saddle Loop	11	3100
85 San Jacinto Peak from the Tramway	11.5	2500
62 San Jacinto Peak via Marion Mountain Trail	12	4600
11 Holcomb Creek	12.75	2200
41 Dollar Lake	13	2400
42 Dry Lake	13	2300
30 Siberia Creek	13	2500
72 Caramba	13.5	3300
50 San Bernardino Peak Divide from Mill Creek	14	5200
58 San Jacinto Peak via Fuller Ridge Trail	15	3600
70 Humber Park–Round Valley Loop	15	3600
48 San Bernardino Peak	16	4700
68 San Jacinto Peak from Humber Park	16	4400
69 Jean Peak and Marion Mountain	16	4600
75 Desert Divide	16.6	2800
52 Dollar Lake Saddle from Mill Creek	20	4500

	Hike	Distance (in miles)	Elevation Gain (in feet)
54	San Gorgonio via Vivian Creek	17	5500
47	San Bernardino Peak Divide from Forsee Creek	18	3700
66	San Jacinto Peak from Idyllwild	19	5200
45	North Fork Meadows	21	4600
43	San Gorgonio via Dollar Lake Saddle	22	4700
44	San Gorgonio via Mine Shaft Saddle	23	4700
49	The Great San Bernardino Divide	30.5	6200

Cool Season

	Hike	Distance (in miles)	Elevation Gain (in feet)
1	Cleghorn Mountain	0.5	100
27	Champion Joshua Tree	1	100
4	Marshall Peak	3	400
88	Lower Palm Canyon	4	200
86	Lykken Loop	4	1000
2	Cajon Mountain	5	300
59	Indian Mountain	5	800
93	Living Desert Zoo and Gardens	5	700
63	Webster Trail	5	1900
83	Cahuilla Mountain	5	800
95	Horsethief Creek	5	900
8	The Pinnacles	6	1000
15	Coxey Creek	6	1400
89	Fern Canyon Loop	6	600
17	Shay Mountain	7	1100
97	Sawmill Trail	8	3700
16	Barrel and Muddy Springs	9	1100
56	Cram and Morton Peaks	9	2800
7	Willow Creek	14	2300
100	Old Santa Rosa	14	2200
98	Rabbit Peak from Coachella Valley	16	6700
90	Jo Pond	17	3800
92	Desert Divide and Palm Canyon	17	2900
91	Palm Canyon Traverse	18	3500
96	Cactus Spring Trail	18	2400
99	Villager and Rabbit Peaks	21	7900

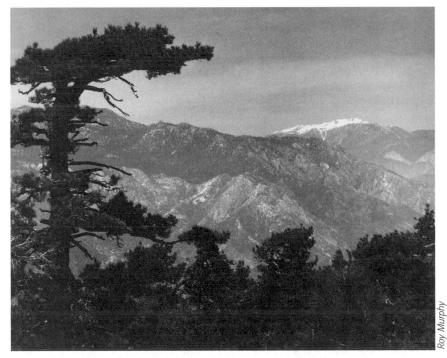

Roy Murphy

San Jacinto Mountains from high in the Santa Rosas, looking north

PART 1

The San Bernardino Mountains

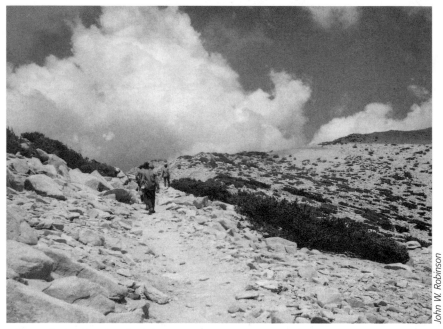

Above timberline on the San Gorgonio Mountain Trail

Natural History of the San Bernardino Mountains

Lay of the Land

From Cajon Pass and the slanted troughs of the great San Andreas Fault, the San Bernardinos rise, rather steeply at first, in chaparral-coated slopes, to the 5000' summits of Cleghorn and Cajon mountains. Eastward from here, for thirty miles, the crest of the San Bernardinos is remarkably uniform. Undulating ridges and tapered hillocks conceal within their folds forested glens and sparkling blue lakes. This is the Crestline–Lake Arrowhead–Running Springs–Big Bear country, the part of the mountains best known to thousands of Southern Californians. Here, among the lakes and streams that form the headwaters of the Mojave River, are summer homes, winter resorts, commercial centers, schools, paved roads by the mile—and only bits and pieces of wilderness.

From Big Bear Lake, the San Bernardinos veer southward and, beyond the deep valley of the upper Santa Ana River, reach their majestic heights in the San Gorgonio Wilderness. Here the hiker and the lover of pristine mountain country can rejoice. Under granite spines hammered up against the sky, lodgepole and limber pines grow sturdy and weather-resistant, tumbling streams flow icy cold, and the thin air is crisp with the chill of elevation. Reigning over all is 11,502' San Gorgonio Mountain—or "Greyback" as it is known to thousands of hikers—the rooftop of Southern California. Early visitors possessed the foresight and initiative to forever preserve this high country in its primitive state.

South from Greyback, the mountains drop abruptly into the deep trench of Mill Creek, rise to rugged Yucaipa Ridge, and finally descend into the San Gorgonio Pass country.

Geologists place the San Bernardino Mountains, as well as the neighboring San Gabriels, in the Transverse Range province—a system of mountain chains that stretch west-to-east, athwart the general northwest-southeast structural grain of California. Like all the Transverse ranges, the San Bernardinos were formed by intensive folding and faulting. The generally smooth summit region of the range—in marked contrast to the rough surface

25

of the San Gabriels—reveals that the San Bernardinos were molded in comparatively recent geologic time. A complex network of faults separates the San Bernardinos from the surrounding landscape. Most pronounced is the great San Andreas Fault, which runs obliquely from northwest to southeast and forms the southern edge of the range. Adjoining the San Andreas is the Mill Creek Fault, which slices through the southern part of the mountains and forms the deep trough of Mill Creek. On the north side of the range, the faultlines, not so clearly evident, appear to be a series of short fracture zones. The largest on this flank is the Helendale Fault, which runs from the Mojave Desert up Cushenbury Canyon to the vicinity of Baldwin Lake. To the east is the Morongo Valley Fault. Other faults slice through the heart of the mountains. The surface rocks of the San Bernardinos are intermixed in great confusion, with granitic types and gneisses predominating, along with quartzites and crystallized limestone.

Plant Life

The forest-and-brush cover of the San Bernardinos shows marked contrast. On the south slopes of the range chaparral predominates. Covering most of the rolling crest of the mountains are lush stands of pine, cedar, and fir. Above 10,000' in the San Gorgonio Wilderness is boreal vegetation, sparse but hardy. Desert-facing slopes on the north and east are primarily pinyon-juniper woodland above and Lower Sonoran vegetation below.

"Nothing seems more hauntingly Californian than the sight and aroma of chaparral drenched in sunlight," wrote a prominent western naturalist. What is chaparral? It is defined as "a dominant, deep-rooted, shrubby vegetation, chiefly evergreen, with leathery, often hard-surfaced leaves." The many-branched shrubs tend to look like miniature trees, and for this reason chaparral has been called "elfin forest." These shrubs can adapt themselves to a wide spectrum of soils, and can exist in terrain and climatic conditions that will support little else. The woodiness of trunks and stems and the thick, small leaves allow chaparral to conserve the moisture they absorb during the short rainy season through the long, hot, rainless summer, so they are ideally suited to Southern California hillsides. Shrubs collectively called chaparral include dozens of species, and many of them are present in the San Bernardinos. The most abundant types here are chamise, scrub oak, manzanita, California holly, and several forms of ceanothus. Hikers generally try to avoid chaparral; indeed, anyone so unfortunate as to become caught in its thorny maze will quickly come to curse it. But those who pay a friendly visit to the elfin forest instead of trying to thrash through it will come to see chaparral in a more favorable light. In bloom, many of the shrubs are sprinkled with colorful flowers. Yucca bursting with fragrant, creamy-white blossoms, ceanothus blooming misty blue or white, California laurel unfolding masses of yellow flowers, wild lilac giving forth its sweet aroma after a spring rain—

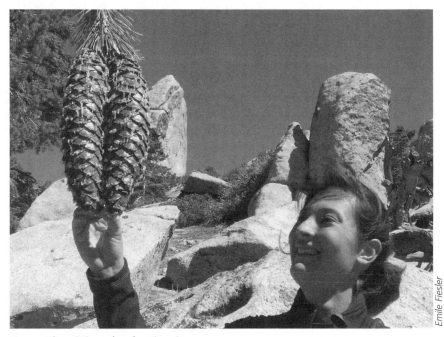

Sugar Pine (*Pinus lambertiana*) cones

these charms await the casual visitor. Chaparral is also valuable as a soil cover; where it has been burned off, rain rushes down the hillsides, causing severe erosion on the slopes and flooding in the canyons and lowlands.

Within the chaparral belt, in the watered canyons, is an association of plants that naturalists call streamside woodland. Lush, verdant growth is the chief characteristic of this habitat. Many varieties of ferns and rushes, and a profusion of flowering herbs grow rich under a green canopy of sycamore, white alder, willow, big-leaf maple, and live oak. After one has slogged for several miles through the elfin forest, reaching this streamside woodland is a special treat—particularly on a warm summer day. The streamside woodlands of Bear and Siberia creeks are particularly delectable.

Amid this ocean of chaparral, nestled on sun-sheltered slopes, are sometimes found islands of bigcone spruce, also known as bigcone Douglas-fir, the lowest-growing conifer in the Southern California mountains. Easily identifiable by its long, horizontal branches and its sparse foliage, this adaptable tree—not an actual spruce—is found from elevations as low as 2000' up into the main mountain forest at 6000' and 7000'.

The crest of the San Bernardinos from Crestline to Big Bear Lake is blessed by a forest as magnificent as any in Southern California. Here grow dense and stately stands of Jeffrey pine, ponderosa pine, sugar pine, Coulter pine, knobcone pine, white fir, and incense-cedar. Adding a beautiful touch of color is the California black oak, its leaves sprouting pink in springtime, light green in summer, and turning a striking yellow in autumn. Beneath ponderosa pine and incense-cedar, we often find Pacific dogwood, and no other forest flower equals the ethereal grace of the dogwood's white blossoms. Walking beneath the canopy of this mountain forest can be a refreshing and enriching experience.

High up in the San Gorgonio Wilderness—on the granite slopes of Greyback and Mount San Bernardino, in the Dry Lake basin—is what naturalists call boreal or subalpine forest. The predominant conifer here is lodgepole pine—tough, cold-resistant, standing erect where sheltered, or twisted and bent where exposed to nature's high-altitude fury. Limber pines, gnarled and ground-hugging, live a marginal existence on the loftiest ridges. The high-altitude chaparral, composed in part of manzanita, snowbrush, bush chinquapin, is rich and green, and waist high. In season, alpine wildflowers burst forth in splashing colors. This is delightful hiking country, a touch of the High Sierra in Southern California. May it ever stay wild.

The backside of the San Bernardinos shows the strong influence of the desert. Here, just over the ridge from the main mountain forest, lying in the "rain shadow" of the range, are extensive stands of pinyon pine and western juniper. Lower down grows that shaggy monarch of the high desert, the Joshua tree. Hard-wooded mountain mahogany thrives on the higher desert-facing slopes. Along Deep Creek and the West Fork of the Mojave grow Fremont cottonwood, desert willow and velvet ash. Mesquite and several varieties of sage are the dominant shrubs below 5000'. This desert slope of the San Bernardinos sees few hikers; this is a shame, for during the cooler months this is an enchanting landscape.

Wildlife

The wildlife of the San Bernardino Mountains is timid, and for the most part, scarce. Man has killed off or driven out many species that once roamed in abundance. Grizzly bears, which were thick in these mountains during pioneer times, have been gone for a century. Black bears—misnamed, for most of them are brown—were once near extinction, but seem to be on the increase. Naturalists estimate that there are around 200–250 in the range. On desert-facing slopes live a handful of statuesque bighorn sheep, extremely shy, seldom seen. There are perhaps fifteen mountain lions in the San Bernardinos. Rare is the hiker who spies one of these big cats romping through the forest, although its large and unmistakable track is sometimes seen on the trail. The most abundant large mammal in the range is the California mule deer. Several thousand head roam the San Bernardinos from top to bottom, feeding on a great variety of plants and sometimes being fed upon by the mountain lion. Smaller mammals include the bobcat, ring-tailed cat, gray fox, coyote, opossum, raccoon, skunk, weasel, and a host of squir-

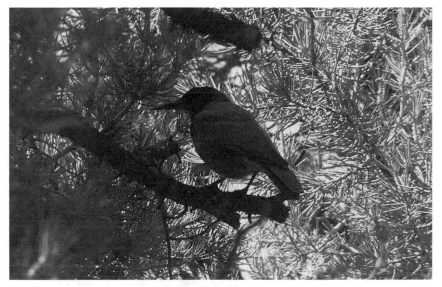

Pinion Jay (*Gymnorhinus cyanocephalus*)

rels and chipmunks. The only creature considered dangerous to man in these mountains is the western rattlesnake, abundant below 6000', sometimes seen up to 8000'. However, most rattlers are not very aggressive and will crawl away if given half a chance.

These, then, are the San Bernardinos—overused yet possessing prime wilderness, smothered with elfin forest below and rich with conifers above, sea-influenced on one side and desert-facing on the other, the highest mountain country in Southern California and some of the most gentle. These are the aspects of the San Bernardinos that have lured visitors into the high country for decades. Come up and sample its delights.

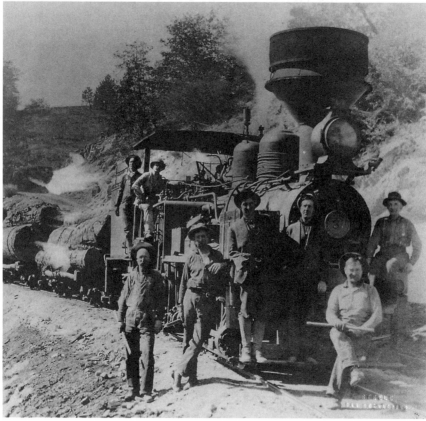

Logging train of the Brookings Lumber Company, 1904

courtesy of Tom Core

Human History of the
San Bernardino Mountains

I only went out for a walk and finally concluded to stay out till sundown, for going out, I found, was really going in.

— John Muir, who visited the
San Bernardino Mountains
in 1896.

Mountains have always held a special significance to humans. They have inspired in us awe and fear and wonder, and filled us with curiosity and longing. They have affected our climate and helped to shape our way of life. They have afforded us livelihood, refuge, pleasure and peace. They have been objects of cherishment and worship. In all, mountains have been a great source of human fulfillment.

The San Bernardino Mountains have been important to us since our ancestors first set foot in Southern California. To Native Americans they were a source of food, water, and materials. Spanish explorers and Californios, the Mexican Californians, sought water and timber. American pioneers expanded the use of water and timber, and added a feverish quest for gold. The mountains continue to entice people to build homes here and find natural areas for recreation, solitude, and relaxation.

A complete history of the San Bernardino Mountains would be a monumental work, covering all of the varied and sometimes hectic human activities in the range. Like the neighboring San Gabriels, the proximity of the San Bernardinos to centers of civilization has resulted in their being swarmed over, dug into, and built upon to a degree equaled by few other mountain ranges in the West. All we have space for here are the highlights of this activity, a sketch to give you a general idea of what humans have done to these mountains.

First Peoples

For untold centuries before the arrival of Europeans, Native Americans lived in and below the San Bernardino Mountains. The mountains provided them acorns, pinyon nuts, berries, and other wild fruits, together with such game as they killed with their bows and arrows or caught in their snares and traps. The mountains were thick with wildlife. Native Americans avoided bears, but relished deer and rabbits, both for their food and their skins. In the mountains they gathered fibers for ropes and baskets, willow splints for arrow shafts, and greasewood for any number of uses.

To make their way through the mountains, Native Americans forged a network of trails. Hunting trails, food-gathering trails, and trading trails crisscrossed much of the range. The most important of these trade routes was the ancient Mojave Trail, which led up the Mojave River into the mountains, up Sawpit Canyon to the crest of the range near today's Monument Peak, and down the south slope via the ridge just west of Devil Canyon. This famous pathway, along with another route through Cajon Pass, was used for centuries by desert Native Americans to trade with peoples living in the San Bernardino Valley and coastal plains.

The Spaniards gave the name *Serrano*—meaning "mountaineer"—to these native peoples of the San Bernardino Mountains. Most of the Serrano villages were located below the south slopes of the range, although some groups apparently lived most of the year well up in the mountains. In the Big Bear region dwelled the Pervetum people, and around Little Bear Valley (now Lake Arrowhead) lived the Kaiwiems. South of the Santa Ana River were villages of the Wanakik or (Pass) Cahuillas, one of the three branches of this widespread Native American group. North and east of the mountains—in the desert and along the Colorado—lived the Mojave people.

Early Explorers

The Spanish soldier Pedro Fages entered the scene in 1772—the first European known to have reached the mountains. Fages was pursuing army deserters from San Diego; he followed them as far as the Colorado Desert. Evidently the desire to do some more exploring seized him, for he turned north and skirted the San Jacinto Mountains by a route Juan Bautista de Anza was to travel two years later. Fages entered the San Bernardino Valley, crossed the mountains in the vicinity of Cajon Pass, and made his way northwest along the south edge of the Mojave Desert to the Tehachapis, the southern San Joaquin Valley, San Luis Obispo, and eventually Monterey.

Fages was followed four years later by the intrepid missionary-explorer-martyr Fray Francisco Hermenegildo Garces, who crossed the San Bernardino Mountains on his way from the lower Colorado River to Mission San Gabriel in 1776. From his diary, it appears that he used the ancient Mojave Trail over the mountains, rather than Cajon Pass. (In 1931, the San

Bernardino County Historical Society erected a monument to mark the point where Garces crossed the crest of the range.)

In a notable 1806 expedition, Fray Jose Zalvidea started from Mission Santa Barbara, explored the southern San Joaquin Valley, crossed the Tehachapis to the desert, and skirted the northern foothills of the San Gabriel and San Bernardino Mountains. Fray Zalvidea and his party entered the latter near the junction of Deep Creek and the Mojave's West Fork, then traversed through Summit Valley and Coyote Canyon into lower Cajon Canyon before continuing on to San Gabriel.

Four years later—on May 20, 1810, the feast day of Saint Bernardino of Siena, a Franciscan preacher of the fifteenth century—a party from Mission San Gabriel set up a temporary chapel in the valley south of the mountains.[1] From this came the name "San Bernardino." This original chapel was evidently short-lived, but in 1819 Spaniards came into the San Bernardino Valley to stay. An *asistencia* of Mission San Gabriel was established southeast of the present city of San Bernardino.

The Spaniards, and a short time later the Californios,[2] soon were engaged in agriculture in the San Bernardino Valley. To bring water to the lands under cultivation, a *zanja* (irrigation ditch) was built from Mill Creek into the valley in 1820. This was the earliest known use of water from the San Bernardino Mountains for irrigation. Timber was taken out also by the Californios. In 1830 mountain hemlock was cut in Mill Creek for use in building the San Bernardino *asistencia*—the earliest known logging in the mountains. Other than taking out water and carrying on some small-scale lumbering, the Spaniards and Californios put the mountains to very little use.

Until the 1840s, only the foothills and low western regions of the San Bernardino Mountains were known to non-natives; the higher country to the east was virtually unexplored. It remained for Benjamin D. Wilson to make known the area now occupied by Big Bear Lake. In the summer of 1845, Wilson, who owned part interest in the Jurupa Rancho (Riverside), led a troop of Mexican cavalry in search of cattle rustlers. Setting out toward the desert, where it was believed the rustlers had headed, Wilson divided his command. Most were sent through Cajon Pass, while Wilson took 22 troopers directly across the mountains. After two days of strenuous travel, Wilson's party reached a wooded valley and a small lake inhabited by scores of grizzly bears. The soldiers formed pairs, and they bagged and skinned eleven bears. Then they continued across the mountains, rejoined the main

---

1 The establishing of this chapel in 1810 is disputed by historians. The original diary reporting its founding has long been lost.

2 This term refers to Mexican Californians. In 1820 Mexico won independence from Spain and by 1823 had established hegemony over California.

party, and surprised the rustlers along the Mojave River. Afterwards, Wilson and his 22 troopers returned home via the mountain lake. Here they lassoed eleven more bears, enough for each man to have a bearskin trophy as a remembrance of the trip. Wilson gave the name *Bear Lake* to the little body of water high in the mountains, and later the grassy basin south of the lake became known as Bear Valley. Years later the name of the body of water Wilson discovered was changed to Baldwin Lake, but the name he gave survives in Big Bear Lake, created when a dam was built at the lower end of Bear Valley in 1884.

The 1840s were watershed years in the history of the mountains. Already mentioned was Wilson's expedition, opening up a part of the range little known before. This was the decade that saw the last of the Native American raids across the mountains, when Wak (or Walkara), a crafty Ute chieftain, led marauding bands through Cajon Pass and over the Mojave Trail, making off with livestock and striking fear in the hearts of rancheros as far as Claremont and Azusa. These raids caused authorities to station soldiers near Cajon Pass. The attacks continued into the 1850s, but on a diminished scale. In 1848 California became part of the United States, and with the coming of the American settlers from the east, the mountains began to receive much more attention.

During these years, the mountains became known by the name they hold today—the San Bernardinos. Thomas Coulter, in his *Notes on Upper California: A Journey from Monterey to the Colorado River in 1832,* published by the Royal Geographical Society of London in 1835, refers to the "great snowy peak of San Bernardino." Coulter, an Irish botanist, is remembered in the name of the Coulter pine. Charles Wilkes' map of 1841 labeled San Bernardino Peak "Mt. Bernardino," and by 1849 most maps showing the mountains used this name or "San Bernardino."

Logging in the San Bernardinos

It was the Mormons, who lived in the San Bernardino Valley from 1851 until 1857, who really opened up the mountains. The Mormon settlers needed lumber for building their town of San Bernardino, and what better place to get this lumber than from the rich stands of pine and cedar in the nearby mountains? Their first efforts were directed toward Mill Creek; here Daniel Sexton built the sawmill in 1852 that gave Mill Creek its name. A second mill was built farther up the creek the following year, known as Mormon Mill. Stumps discovered years later revealed that lumbering was undertaken as far up-canyon as the site of present-day Fallsvale, well up under the shoulder of San Gorgonio Mountain.

Mill Creek met the Mormons' lumber needs for several months, but soon their eyes turned to the much richer stands of timber on the mountain crest to the north. But first a road would have to be built up the steep south slopes of the range. This was accomplished through back-breaking efforts in 1853, by "every man leaving his family in camp and freely laboring and camping upon the road incessantly until finished." This first road onto the crest of the San Bernardinos climbed directly up Hot Springs (later Waterman) Canyon and gave access to Seeley and Huston flats, then heavily timbered. Charles Crisman built the first sawmill here within ten days of the road's completion, dragging up an engine and boiler for this small, portable operation. The first major sawmill on the mountain crest was erected by the brothers David and Wellington Seely in the summer of 1853; they used waterpower from the creek flowing through Seely Flat. Oxen hauled the cut wood down to San Bernardino. By the middle of 1854 the Mormons had six mills operating in the San Bernardino Mountains—four on the mountain crest and two on Mill Creek. Most of the lumber was used in San Bernardino, but some was hauled as far away as Los Angeles.

The Mormons returned to Utah in 1857, but the mountain sawmills remained, and more were built in ensuing years. Strawberry Valley, Grass Valley, Little Bear Valley (later Lake Arrowhead), Hooks Creek, Twin Peaks, Green Valley, Snow Valley, Big Bear, Holcomb Valley and Barton Flats all were the scene of lumbering operations, some of them continuing into recent years. Most ambitious were the activities of the Brookings Lumber Company at Fredalba, near today's Running Springs, in operation from 1898 until 1910. Robert Brookings built a narrow gauge logging railroad network that gave access to most of the timber between Heaps Peak and Arrowbear Lake—quite an expanse of mountain country (see photo on page 30). Remnants of this turn-of-the-century operation are still visible.

Southern California's Goldrush

Timber was the first magnet that lured non-natives into the San Bernardino Mountains; gold was the second. The precious metal was reportedly found in the mountains as early as 1857 and there was some prospecting activity in 1859, but not until William F. Holcomb made his famous discovery in Holcomb Valley in 1860 was there a real gold rush. The story goes that Holcomb and a companion named Ben Chouteau, members of a prospecting party in Bear Valley, crossed the ridge that separates the waters of the Santa Ana River from those of the Mojave River during a hunting trip, and shot two bears. Next day they returned to secure the animals, and in addition to obtaining bear meat they discovered something much more thrilling—gold! Within a week the entire Holcomb party had moved into the gold-laden basin—later known as Holcomb Valley—and were feverishly digging for placer gold. The news of the discovery spread to San Bernardino, and by early July Holcomb Valley was swarming with prospectors, who were making $5 to $10 a day. A boom town sprung up in short order; the miners named it Belleville, in honor of little Belle Van Dusen, whose mother had

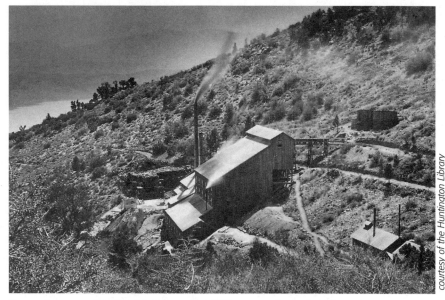

courtesy of the Huntington Library

Rare photograph of Gold Mountain Mill in operation, circa 1910

furnished a flag for a patriotic occasion. More gold was discovered across the ridge in Bear Valley, and by the fall of 1860 the entire mountain region was overrun with gold seekers.

The original route to the mines was by wagon road from San Bernardino to the mouth of Santa Ana Canyon, then by steep pack trail up the Santa Ana River to Seven Oaks and over the ridge into Bear Valley. Bringing in provisions by this route was difficult and expensive, so the miners subscribed $1500, which they gave to a Mr. Van Dusen to build a new wagon road. Van Dusen wisely decided that the south slope of the range below Bear Valley was too steep and rugged for such a road; instead he built his road northwesterly from Holcomb Valley down to the Mojave River, then southwest to near the head of Cajon Pass, where it met the toll road through the pass into the San Bernardino Valley just completed by John Brown. By this roundabout route, all types of supplies were transported to the mines.

Through most of the 1860s, mining activities involving hundreds of men continued in Holcomb and Bear valleys. At one time the population in Holcomb Valley alone is said to have reached 2000. These were years of stormy excitement and controversy. Ruffians and outlaws came in large numbers, and during the Civil War, Southern sympathizers were vocal and active. As many as 40 men and probably many more met violent deaths during this frenzied period. But gradually the placer gold gave out and the miners drifted away to new diggings elsewhere in the west. By 1870 Belleville was a ghost town and Holcomb Valley's hectic era was history.

Although the placer gold was gone, many quartz-gold prospects remained, hidden in canyons and hillsides throughout the Holcomb Valley–Bear Valley area. The last three decades of the 1800s saw the development of many of these hard-rock prospects—the Osborne Mine northeast of Holcomb Valley, the Ozier on John Bull Flat, the Rose Mine southeast of Baldwin Lake, the Santa Fe group in Blackhawk Canyon, and, most productive of all, Lucky Baldwin's Doble Mine on Gold Mountain. Gold was mined and milled at these and other prospects well into this century.

Blue Gold

Water was the third lure that brought outsiders into the San Bernardino Mountains. The streams gushing down from the high country had been utilized for domestic purposes and irrigation since settlers had first made homes in the San Bernardino Valley. But most of the water was wasted, flowing out to sea during the wetter months, and not available during the hot months when many of the streams dried up. The possibility of using Bear Valley as a storage reservoir was brought to public attention in 1880, when a state engineer's survey said the basin was one of the best sites for such a reservoir in Southern California. In 1883 the founders of the new colony of Redlands incorporated the Bear Valley Land and Water Company, intent upon impounding water in a mountain reservoir for use on the newly developed valley land. A single-arch, stone-and-cement dam was completed at a cost of $75,000 the following year; thus was born Big Bear Lake. Although the mountain lake was now reality and the dam (to the surprise of many

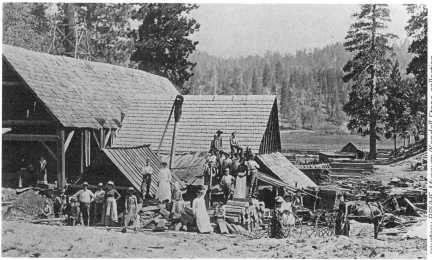

The Talmadge Sawmill in Little Bear Valley (now under the waters of Lake Arrowhead) — 1870s

engineers) held, the water company was flooded with a mass of litigation over water rights that lasted for decades. In 1910–11 a second, stronger dam was constructed just below the original one; this is the dam the highway crosses today, holding back a lake eight miles long, containing 72,000 acre-feet of water.

Lake Arrowhead was formed in much the same way. In 1891 a group of Ohio businessmen organized the Arrowhead Reservoir Company, and two years later began construction of a dam across Little Bear Creek. The dam was completed in 1908, and tunnels were dug to divert the waters from their natural flow (northward) to the San Bernardino Valley. But a mass of litigation was involved here too. The state supreme court doomed the irrigation project by ruling that water could not be diverted from one watershed to another. But Little Bear Lake remained, to be renamed Lake Arrowhead in 1922.

During this era a number of toll roads were built into the mountains. The first ones were the Daley Road up Twin Creek Canyon, built in 1859, and the Cajon Pass Toll Road constructed by John Brown two years later. During the 1890s four new ones appeared—the Bear Valley, City Creek Canyon, Devils Canyon, and Arrowhead Reservoir Company toll roads. On the desert side the Johnson and Cushenbury grades were gouged out and another route opened into the high country. Then came the most famous road of all, the Rim of the World Highway (State Highway 18), 101 miles long, completed in 1915.

Today's Gold: Recreation

With the roads came people, and with people arose the fourth lure of the mountains, recreation. At first there were cabins, then hotels and stores and saloons. Gus Knight Jr. built the first mountain resort at Big Bear Lake in the 1890s. Pine Knot was the first lakeside community here. Down in the canyon of the Santa Ana River was Seven Oaks, a popular tent camp in the '90s. In the 1920s Lake Arrowhead became a resort community, and subdivision for residential purposes began. Then came the development of Crestline, Lake Gregory, Running Springs, Green Valley, and many more centers of civilization in the high country. The mountains were being overrun by people.

Fortunately, humankind includes those who work to protect and preserve as well as those who might pillage and destroy. By 1890 it was evident to many farsighted people that the San Bernardino Mountains needed federal protection. Even those with myopic vision could see that reckless cutting of timber was destroying the mountain watershed. As a result of strong pressure from conservation-minded citizens, President Benjamin Harrison signed an act creating the San Bernardino Forest Reserve, on February 25, 1893. In 1898 the first rangers were assigned to the reserve and a patrol sys-

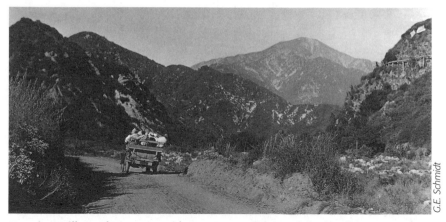

Entering Mill Creek Canyon, with San Bernardino Peak in the distance – 1915

tem was established. Unfortunately, large areas of the high country were already in private ownership and outside the jurisdiction of the Forest Service. But the lands within the forest reserve were zealously guarded, and, starting about 1902, burned areas were reforested. In 1908 the San Bernardino Forest Reserve was joined with the Angeles and the designation was changed from forest reserve to national forest. This union lasted until 1925, when San Bernardino National Forest again became a separate entity. In 1931 the highest and most primitive part of the mountains was set aside as the San Gorgonio Primitive Area (since 1964, the San Gorgonio Wilderness), to be forever preserved in its natural state.

Today, the San Bernardinos receive annually about fifteen million visitors, making them one of the most heavily used mountain regions in the nation. With this many people motoring, sightseeing, picnicking, camping, horseback riding, boating, skiing, and hiking in the mountains, nature is hardpressed to hold its own.

Even areas considered inviolate face pressures generated by the people explosion. During the early 1960s, commercial skiing interests waged a determined and almost successful effort to "open up" the heart of the San Gorgonio Wilderness to roads, resorts and ski lifts. Conservationists, led by the Defenders of the San Gorgonio Wilderness, barely won that battle. Now the problem is not skiers but hikers—too many of them swarming over wilderness trails and into campgrounds. To save the wilderness from the perils of overuse, the Forest Service in 1971 instituted the wilderness permit system. Permits are now rationed in most wilderness areas, allowing only a limited number of people to enter the area at one time.

Regardless of the history, the future of these mountains rests with the people who frequent them. They are the ultimate guardians of Nature's handiwork.

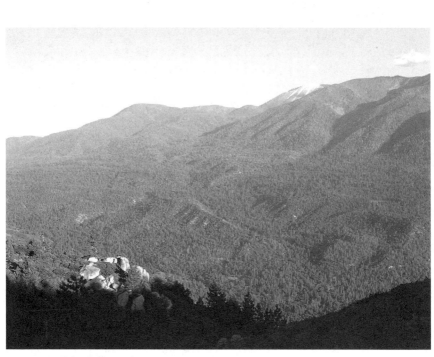

San Gorgonio (Hike 44)

CLEGHORN MOUNTAIN

Hike Length: 0.5 mile round trip; 100' elevation gain
Difficulty: Easy
Season: November–May
Topo map: *Cajon* (7.5')

Features

Cajon Pass, the deep cleft separating the San Gabriel from the San Bernardino mountains, is an historic gateway from the Mojave Desert to the Southern California coastal lowlands. Native Americans, explorers, trappers, traders, and settlers were the pioneers who journeyed through the Cajon, and today the pass is the route of major highway and railroad arteries. Geologists say Cajon Pass was formed as a result of an overlapping of the east end of the San Gabriel Mountains with the west end of the San Bernardinos, caused by the earth-twisting movements of the San Andreas Fault, which cuts right through Cajon Canyon.

This trip takes you up the west end of the San Bernardinos for a bird's-eye panorama of this gateway to the Southland, with the abrupt northeast face of the San Gabriel Mountains as an imposing backdrop. Few other vantage points offer such a view of this historic cut in the mountains. The trip is through rather scraggly chaparral, on fire road and firebreak all the way, so it is best done on a cool winter or spring day, when the chaparral is blooming and fragrant, and the air is crisp and clean-washed.

The Cleghorn Ridge Road (2N47) has been upgraded and is now a popular route for recreational vehicles, especially on weekends. With a four-wheel-drive (4WD) vehicle, you can now drive to a point just 0.25 mile from Cleghorn Mountain's summit, which has turned this once-long hike into a short walk. In winter, with snow on the road, this trip becomes a longer hike.

Cleghorn Mountain—and Cleghorn Ridge, Cleghorn Pass and Cleghorn Canyon—were named for Matthew Cleghorn and his son John, who leased this western tip of the San Bernardinos for timber-cutting back in the 1870s. They must have been thorough; there is little timber left here today. Before the Civil War, the area was used by thieves who drove thousands of stolen horses and mules from Southern California for resale in Utah. In 1927, the Elliot Ranch was built on a 30 acre homestead.

The 2003 Old Fire tore through these hills. The burn was so severe that it closed the roads for two years, but work crews have now restored access.

Description

From Interstate 15 (freeway), 17 miles up from San Bernardino, turn right (northeast) onto State Highway 138 and continue 4 miles. At mile marker

19.5 you reach the road leading left to Summit Railroad Station (the point of the real Cajon Pass); on your right (south) a sign indicates ELLIOTT. Turn and follow this fair dirt road 3N22 southwest, going straight ahead where a road drops left, to a second junction, 1.5 miles from Highway 138. If snow is on the road or you want a moderate hike, start walking here (**GPS SB01A**), going left (east) up Cleghorn Ridge Road (2N47), 7 miles round trip with 1300 elevation gain. Otherwise, turn left at the second junction and drive up 2N47 just 3.5 miles to a clearing immediately west of Cleghorn's rounded summit. Park here (**GPS SB01B**) and walk up then left through low brush to the top, 0.25 mile.

From the 5333' summit, look northwest at the jumbled ridgeline that forms the summit of the Cajon. First you see the Santa Fe Railroad tracks, built in 1885, passing Summit Station—the low point of the pass. 1.5 miles beyond (north of) Summit Station is a shallow defile, which was the route of the historic Old Spanish Trail, used by explorers, hunters, trappers, traders, and soldiers since the 1770s. Today only a seldom-used dirt road crosses here. Two miles beyond the old Spanish route, winding up the hillside and most obvious of all, is the Interstate 15 freeway, crossing the divide at Cajon Summit. Farther west from Interstate 15 you can see the old highway crossing, the remains of Sanford's old wagon road put through in 1855, and State Highway 138 leading to Palmdale. Perhaps no other pass in the West has been so cut up by humans: and you see it all from Cleghorn Mountain.

Return the way you came. An alternate route, requiring a car shuttle, is to drop southeast down the firebreak to the fire road at Cleghorn Pass (see Hike 2).

It is also possible to drive or hike down 2N47 from the junction of Cleghorn Road with Interstate 15. The fair dirt road switchbacks down the steep mountainside, giving an odd feeling of remoteness within a stones throw of the freeway. This variation descends 3.8 miles and 900 feet to the freeway (**GPS SB01C**).

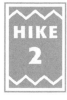

CAJON MOUNTAIN

Hike Length: 5 miles round trip; 300' elevation gain
Difficulty: Easy
Season: November–May
Topo map: *Cajon* (7.5')

Features

Cajon Mountain (5310') towers over the lower end of the Cajon Pass area, and its summit offers a sweeping panorama of the great fault-carved passage through the mountains. From here you can see the San Andreas Fault, its strange slanting ridges and twisted rock formations all bearing in a northwest-southeast direction. Directly below is the Blue Cut, where Cajon Canyon narrows to a gorge and crosses the fault. The view beyond is equally grand, with Mt. San Antonio (Old Baldy) and the cluster of high peaks at the east end of the San Gabriels looming massive and grayish.

This trip is all on fire road, shaded part of the way by California black oak, bigcone spruce and sugar pine. In the winter and early spring, the eastern peaks of the San Gabriels are dazzling in their mantle of whiteness, and the foothills are velvet-green.

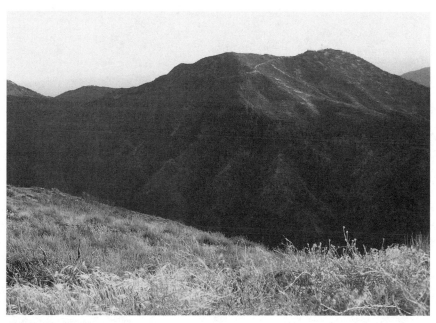

Cajon Mountain at sunset

Description

From Interstate 15 (freeway) turn right (northeast) onto State Highway 138. Follow this road northeast, east through Summit Valley, and south along the West Fork of the Mojave River 11 miles to the clearly marked exit for Cleghorn Road just beyond mile marker 138 SBD 26.18. Note that this Cleghorn Road is Forest Service Road 2N49, not to be confused with the other Cleghorn Road, 2N47, coming up from Interstate 15 (see Hike 1). Turn right (west) and drive past group camps. Cleghorn turns into a poor dirt fire road (2N49) 0.9 mile from the highway, then passes an unlocked gate after another 0.2 mile. Continue 5.4 more miles, passing Cleghorn Pass, to a junction with Cajon Mountain Road, on your right (west), 6.5 miles from Highway 138. Park outside the locked gate (**GPS SB02**). The Cajon Mountain Road gate is sometimes open, in which case one can skip the hike and drive to the lookout with a 4WD vehicle.

Proceed past the locked gate, following Cajon Mountain Road through an open forest of black oak, big-cone Douglas-fir, and sugar pine, as it descends to a saddle, then climbs to the 5310' summit of Cajon Mountain and its fire-lookout tower, 2.5 miles. Much of this area burned in the Willow fire of 1999 and then again in the Old fire of 2003. Enjoy the superb panorama, then return the same way.

HEART ROCK

Hike Length: 2 miles round trip; 300' elevation gain
Difficulty: Easy
Season: All year
Topo map: *Silverwood Lake* (7.5')

Features

Seeley Creek descends the north slope of the San Bernardinos, from its source west of Crestline to Miller Canyon, and eventually into the Mojave River. This short, delightful forest walk follows a one-mile stretch of the bubbling creek under a canopy of very tall Jeffrey pines, incense-cedars, and black oaks. You end up alongside two limpid pools with a natural waterslide between. Nearby is Heart Rock, with a heart-shaped hole in the middle through which water sometimes splashes. For an introduction to the San Bernardinos, you can do no better than this magnificent forest stroll.

Thoughtless people leave their litter beside the pools on the creek. If you bring a trash bag and carry some of it out, you'll help keep the creek beautiful for all of us.

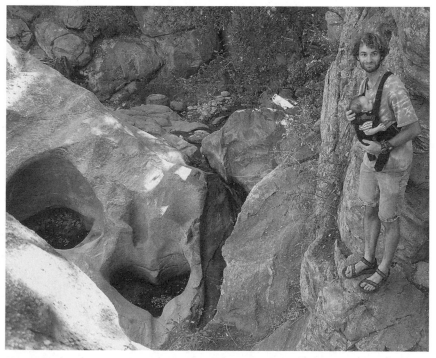

Heart Rock

Description

From Crestline, take State Highway 138 northwest, down to the Camp Seeley entrance road at mile marker 138 SBD 35.00, 1.5 miles. Turn left, then left again just outside the gate to Camp Seeley, and follow the narrow paved road to a parking area on your right, marked with a metal pole with 4W07 (the trail number) on it, 0.4 mile from the highway (**GPS SB03**).

Walk down the broad trail as it descends north, through a shady forest of Jeffrey pine and incense-cedar, just above the creek. After 0.25 mile, your pathway climbs a slight rise and forks as Seeley Creek abruptly drops. To your right, a short walk gets you to a rocky outcropping directly above Seeley Creek, where you look down on Heart Rock with its hole in the middle. Return to the main trail and follow it steeply down to the creek. Here, deep in the forest, are two pools with a natural waterslide between.

Return the same way.

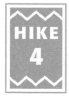

MARSHALL PEAK

HIKE 4

Hike Length: 3 miles round trip; 400' elevation gain
Difficulty: Easy
Season: October–May
Topo map: *San Bernardino North* (7.5')

Features

After a storm, when the sky is washed clean and the high mountains are glistening in their snow mantle, walk the short distance to Marshall Peak for an inspiring panorama. Overlooking the wrinkled foothills of the San Bernardinos, Marshall Peak offers a superb panorama of the valley, with the east-end high country of the San Gabriels, the San Gorgonio Wilderness, and the distant San Jacintos looming as lofty backdrops.

This trip, through chaparral all the way and mostly on fire road, ends with a short scramble up a firebreak to the rounded summit.

This trip is in the heart of the fire damage caused by the 2003 Old Fire. Only blackened core branches of manzanita and chaparral remain on the denuded landscape. This is an excellent trip for witnessing the devastation caused by a major forest fire and to observe the regeneration in the years to

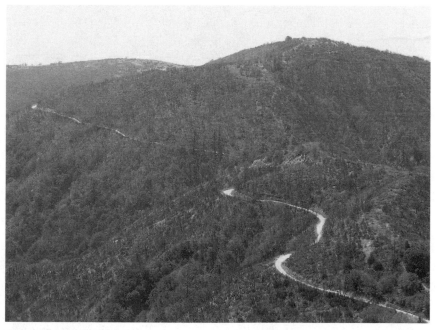

Marshall Peak fire road

come. The following spring after the fire, patches of green grass already covered the surrounding slopes. By 2005, the hills are thick with new brush sprouting amidst the blackened tentacles of manzanita.

Description

From the Rim of the World Highway (State Highway 18), 9.5 miles up from Highland Avenue in San Bernardino and just past mile marker 14.80, turn left into a huge turnout (**GPS SB04**). A gate on the south side marks the entrance to fire road 2N40. Park outside the gate without blocking the entrance. The gate is sometimes open, in which case, this hike can become a short drive if you prefer.

Follow the fair dirt fire road south along the ridge, traversing around the east slope of two small bumps, to its intersection with the Cloudland Forest fire road, 1.3 miles. From the intersection, continue 0.1 mile up the road to a firebreak next to a fence on the right, and scramble 0.1 more miles up the firebreak to the top (**GPS SB04A**) (or stay on the main road, which also winds around to the summit).

Return the same way. An option is to descend the Cloudland Forest fire road southeast to its junction with the Rim of the World Highway (State Highway 18) just above Inspiration Point, 3 miles. This would require a 5-mile car shuttle.

ARROWHEAD PEAK

Hike Length: 6 miles round trip; 1400' elevation gain
Difficulty: Moderate
Season: All year
Topo map: *San Bernardino North* (7.5')

Features

Above San Bernardino, as if branded onto the mountainside, is a near-perfect figure of an arrowhead pointing downward. Even more amazing, this nature-patterned landmark points directly to hot springs bubbling out of the mountain. Although not as distinct as it once was, the Arrowhead can still be readily observed by anyone starting up the Rim of the World Highway (State Highway 18) from San Bernardino.

Naturalists have studied this unique monument to discover how it was formed. They have found that, 18 inches under the surface of the Arrowhead, there is granite, so that only shallow-rooted mountain sage and a few other bedrock species of a light grey-green color can grow here. The soil outside the Arrowhead is deeper, and it sustains greasewood and other darker shrubs. Hence the distinct color difference, forming the outline of the downward-pointing symbol.

The Arrowhead is the subject of a host of Native American legends, and a few from more modern times. No other natural landmark in the San Bernardino Mountains has in the past been so regarded with awe and wonder. The most repeated tale is the Cahuilla legend: Long ago the Cahuillas dwelt in lands far to the east. Although of a peace-loving disposition, they were constantly harassed by warlike neighbors. At last they could no longer endure their persecutions, so they called upon the God of Peace to help them find a new home where they could dwell in solitude. Being a gentle people, they were looked upon with favor by the Great Spirit. They were told to travel westward and watch for a fiery arrow in the sky, which would direct them to their new homeland. The Cahuillas started on their journey, and one moonless night there shot across the heavens a blazing arrow. The arrow finally came down upon a mountainside where the shaft was consumed by fire but the head embedded itself on the slope. The Native Americans aroused themselves from their camp and journeyed hastily to the still-glowing arrowhead. Here they lived happily ever after.

Directly below the Arrowhead are boiling hot springs, long used to bring relief to victims of rheumatism and other similar afflictions. Dr. David N. Smith was first to develop those hot springs; in 1863 he built a few cabins here and two years later he erected a hotel. This hotel was later destroyed by fire, as were two successors, the last one in 1937. Today the hotel and grounds are international headquarters for the Campus Crusade for Christ.

Unfortunately Campus Crusade for Christ has closed the lower end of the Arrowhead Trail. So you must do this trip from above, hiking down from the Rim of the World Highway (State Highway 18), enjoying far-reaching views of the abrupt south front of the range. You're walking through chaparral all the way, so do it on a cool day. As in Hike 4, this area was in the heart of the 2003 Old Fire. It is an excellent location for viewing the effects of a major forest fire. The Rim of the World Highway was closed until August 2005 by slides resulting from erosion after the fire. The route is becoming badly over-grown, so long pants, boots, and even gloves are helpful.

Description

From San Bernardino, drive up Waterman Avenue, which becomes the Rim of the World Highway (State Highway 18). As you drive through town, you will see a signed historical marker on the right next to an athletic field. The marker offers a good view of the Arrowhead and an explanation of the legends behind the landmark. Continue up Highway 18 1.6 miles beyond the Crestline junction and park in a prominent clearing to the right of the highway at mile marker 19.45 (**GPS SB05**).

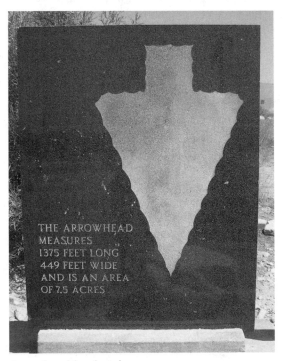

Arrowhead landmark

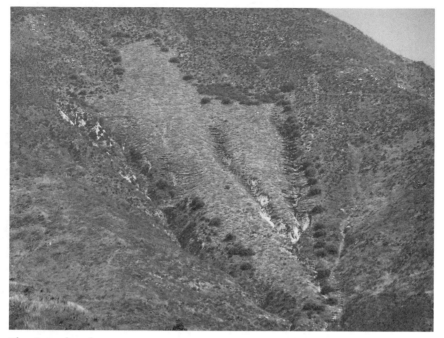

The Arrowhead

Walk past the gate on the west end of the lot and follow the trail, eroded and heavily overgrown in places (it's an old fire road), as it switchbacks down to a saddle north of Arrowhead Peak. Your trail then climbs along the west shoulder of a ridge, high above Waterman Canyon, drops again, then climbs over the summit of Arrowhead Peak (4237'). Here your views are magnificent, over the abrupt south rampart of the mountains, down across the often mist-shrouded San Bernardino Valley, and eastward to snow-streaked San Bernardino Peak and the Yucaipa Ridge.

Hikers who want a moderate, view-rich walk should turn back here. If you desire a close-up view of the Arrowhead and don't mind a long uphill trudge on the return, continue down the trail, which drops steeply in places, to the top of the Arrowhead, a mile farther. Remember, the lower end of the trail is closed, so after you've examined this unique geological feature, return back up the way you came.

DEEP CREEK HOT SPRINGS

HIKE 6

Hike Length:	3 miles round trip; 700' elevation gain
Difficulty:	Easy
Season:	All year
Topo map:	*Lake Arrowhead* (7.5')
Permit:	Permission of land owner required

Features

Deep Creek, on the north slope of the mountains, boasts the only genuine hot springs in the San Bernardinos. As many as 20 hikers bathe in the three warm pools beside the cold creek on winter weekends. During the summer, Deep Creek offers swimming holes and sandy beaches near the springs. Overnight camping is disallowed at the hot springs, but you may camp at Bowen Ranch. Please protect the hot springs: do not bring glass and make a special effort to leave the place cleaner than you found it.

Description

From Interstate 15, 6 miles north of Cajon Pass, turn right (east) at the Hesperia turn-off. Proceed through Hesperia on Main Street for 7.2 miles, then bear left (east) on Rock Springs Road where Main Street curves south. Cross the dry bed of the Mojave River and follow Rock Springs Road east to its end, 10.2 miles from the freeway. Go left (north) 0.5 mile, then right (east) on Roundup Way. Follow the latter 4.4 miles, then turn right (south) onto the good dirt Bowen Ranch Road. Proceed up the latter, going right at a junction with a huge BLM sign at 2.1 miles, and right again in 1.9 miles at another junction with the Oak Springs Road, to Bowen Ranch, on the left 5.4 miles from Roundup Way (**GPS SB06**). After heavy rains, Rock Springs Road is sometimes washed out at the Mojave River. The next river crossing further north is on Bear Valley Road. After crossing the river on Bear Valley, drive east to Central, then turn right and drive south for 3.4 miles to reach Roundup. Turn left and proceed to Bowen Ranch Road.

You must stop at the ranch house, register, and pay a modest fee. Camping is allowed 0.5 mile beyond the ranch house. The trail begins at road's end atop a hill. You descend south, pass through a gate when you enter Forest Service land, and veer left, then right down a wash. You traverse a ridge, then drop steeply down to Deep Creek, 1.5 miles from the start. The hot springs are across the creek and just downstream.

The hottest pool is enclosed in rocks 20 feet above the creek. Luke-warm pools are below, separated from the creek by a constructed rock barrier.

Return the way you came. Remember, it's all uphill on the way back.

WILLOW CREEK

Hike Length: 14 miles round trip; 2300' elevation gain
Difficulty: Strenuous
Season: September–June
Topo maps: *Lake Arrowhead* (7.5')

Features

Willow Creek, a tributary of Deep Creek, drains the Rock Camp area north of Lake Arrowhead. It runs full after spring rains, but reduces to a trickle by mid-summer. The 63,000-acre Willow Fire of September 1999 burned over much of this drainage, but the chaparral below is fast growing back. The first two miles of this trip follow an off-road vehicle track. The long section down Willow Creek is difficult to follow in several places.

Description

From State Route 173, 5 miles north of Lake Arrowhead to Rock Camp Forest Service Station (no services). At the time of this writing, 173 is closed for repairs from fire damage between the northern part of Lake Arrowhead and Grass Valley Road. An alternate approach from the west on Highway 18 involves driving northeast on Highway 189 for about 3 miles to Grass Valley Road, then continuing north on Grass Valley Road another 4 miles to its junction with Highway 173 just north of the closure. Rock Camp is 0.2 mile north of Grass Valley Road.

The gate to Rock Camp is open from 9:30 A.M. to 6:00 P.M. at the time of this writing, so you may prefer to park in the lot across the highway from Rock Camp (**GPS SB07**). Walk across to Rock Camp and follow signs for the Interpretive Trail (formerly called Metate Trail).

Pass through the gate and follow the trail, well-worn by off-road vehicle tracks, northeastward down to a junction with the North Shore Trail, coming in to your right, 1.5 miles. Follow your Metate Trail northward to a junction with Forest Road 3N34, 0.5 mile. Turn right and follow 3N34 down across Willow Creek. 50 yards east of Willow Creek, look for an indistinct trail leading left, down the east slope of the Willow Creek drainage. Here you leave off-road vehicles and civilization behind and enter a wilderness. Your trail, faint in some places, distinct in others, descends northward, staying well above the churning waters of Willow Creek, winding up and down and around several side canyons. You reach a junction with the Pacific Crest Trail, on the south slope of Deep Creek Canyon. Turn left and follow the PCT downstream 2 miles to Deep Creek Hot Springs. Return the way you came, or climb to Bowen Ranch, which requires a long car shuttle (see Hike 6).

The trip can be shortened by driving north on Highway 173 past Rock Camp to 3N34, then following the dirt road east to Willow Creek.

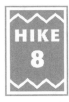

THE PINNACLES

Hike Length: 6 miles round trip; 1000' elevation gain
Difficulty: Moderate
Season: November–May
Topo map: *Lake Arrowhead* (7.5')

Features

The Pinnacles are an imposing stack of jumbo, weathered granite boulders cutting high over the badlands terrain on the desert-facing slope of the San Bernardinos.

Description

From State Route 173, drive 6 miles north of Lake Arrowhead to the Arrowhead Rifle Range on the left side. Park off the highway on the right (east) side (**GPS SB08**). At the time of this writing, 173 is closed north of Lake Arrowhead for repairs from fire damage; see Hike 7 for aternative directions.

Your trail begins at an opening in the fence, bounded by two wooden posts, just before (south of) the entrance to the rifle range. The trail hugs the south edge of the fenced range. Follow it northwest as it and ascends a boulder-strewn ridge. Continue northwest through scrawny chaparral and around large boulders, looking for ducks, to the foot of the main ridge.

Climb the left (south) side of the boulder-stacked ridge, going around the left side of the high point you see (class 3 climbing—use caution). At the top of the ridge, you will see the summit about 0.25 mile beyond; work your way over and around the boulders to it.

Descend the same way, making certain your general direction is southeast. (Climbers have descended the wrong way, taking hours to go through this badlands country back to camp.)

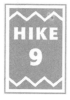

LITTLE BEAR CREEK

HIKE 9

Hike Length: 5 miles round trip; 800' elevation gain
Difficulty: Moderate
Season: All year
Topo map: *Lake Arrowhead* (7.5')

Features

The canyon of Little Bear Creek—just east of Lake Arrowhead—was a delight to visit. A small stream glides and dances over water-tempered boulders, shaded by magnificent Jeffrey and sugar pines and incense-cedars. Ferns and grasses grew lush along the banks. Just over the ridge, civilization seems far away. The 2003 Old Fire incinerated almost everything on this trip. Consider this a unique opportunity to witness both the complete devastation of a major forest fire and the regeneration of the forest.

The trip descends from North Shore Campground, just east of Lake Arrowhead, to visit this verdant sanctuary and observe the regrowth.

Description

From State Highway 173, 2.8 miles northeast of the junction with Highway 189 at Lake Arrowhead Village, turn right (east) onto Hospital Road. Follow the latter 0.25 mile to campground entrance, opposite the hospital. If you park in the campground you must pay the day-use fee. You can park free outside the campground, but not in the hospital parking lot without permission. The campground amazingly escaped the 2003 Old Fire. As of this writing, the campground is open between May 15 and September 30.

Your trail (3W12) begins at the extreme eastern end of the campground by the Forest Service sign for the Rim of the World Scenic Trail (**GPS SB09**). Follow the trail downhill, crossing a dirt road, into the shady recess of Little Bear Creek. Now the trees are charred but the vegetation in the streambed is rapidly regrowing. The path follows the left (north) bank of the trickling creek, climbs 50' over a ridge to shortcut a horseshoe bend, and continues alongside the stream, then makes an abrupt right turn and crosses the creek to Hooks Creek Road (2N26Y), 2.5 miles from the start.

You can return uphill the way you came, or have someone pick you up at your meeting with Forest Service road 2N26Y near the trailhead for Hike 10 (**GPS SB09A**).

DEEP CREEK

Hike Length:	5 miles round trip; 500' elevation gain
Difficulty:	Moderate
Season:	All year
Topo map:	*Lake Arrowhead, Butler Peak* (both 7.5')

Features

Deep Creek cuts an impressive swath through the north-slope country of the San Bernardinos. The creek and its numerous tributaries drain most of the mountain region from Lake Arrowhead almost to Big Bear. Although not so named, Deep Creek is really the east fork of the Mojave River. Its abundant waters flow year-round, sometimes becoming a raging torrent in stormy times.

About midway between its headwaters and its junction with the West Fork of the Mojave, Deep Creek runs through rugged, rock-ribbed terrain. Its waters tumble and cascade among huge boulders, here and there pausing briefly in limpid pools. This is the Devils Hole country; the Devils Hole itself is in a narrow chasm just east of the creek.

This is a trip for those who like to explore deep canyons and rushing creeks. It's easy walking on the slopes above Deep Creek on a section of the Pacific Crest Trail. Bring your fishing rod, for trout linger in some of the pools.

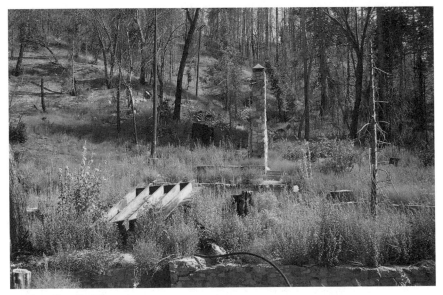

Cedar Glen fire damage

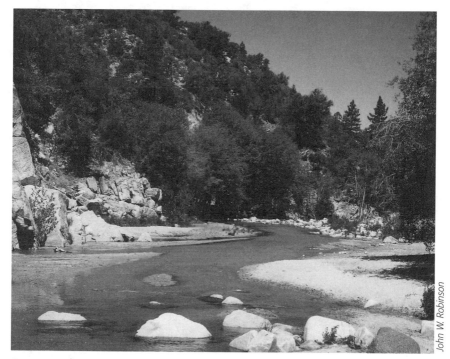

Deep Creek

The 2003 Old Fire devastated the forest on the southern end of this trip and many homes in Cedar Glen. The Pacific Crest Trail (PCT) is intact but the forest has been burned to about 1.5 miles north of where the PCT crosses Deep Creek. The steel bridge across Deep Creek was partially destroyed when a large burning pine tree crushed the east end of the bridge.

Description

From Highway 173 1.6 miles northeast of the junction with Highway 189 at Lake Arrowhead Village, drive east on Hook Creek Road through the village of Cedar Glen for 2.3 miles to a gate at Forest Service Road 2N26Y. Continue 0.8 mile down the windy one-lane road (with speed bumps!) and cross Little Bear Creek. Continue 0.1 mile on a good dirt road to a signed fork where 2N26Y meets a sharp bend in 3N34. Trail 3W12 from North Shore campground (Hike 9) ends close to this point. Stay left at the junction on 3N34. Cross the creek again and make a right turn at 3N34C after 0.2 mile. Pass another gate (**GPS SB10**) and proceed 0.3 mile to the Splinters Cabin trailhead where the hike begins. If either gate is locked, park outside and walk from the gate, taking care not to block access to the gate or to private property on Hook Creek Road.

Take the trail that leaves the north end of the parking area. You ford Little Bear Creek and reach the Pacific Crest Trail in 0.25 mile. Follow the PCT north as it climbs and then contours above Deep Creek, shaded by numerous live oaks. You then descend gently, matching the gradient of Deep Creek, and pass the confluence of Holcomb Creek, its waters churning in from the east. Continuing north on the PCT, you descend open slopes 150 feet above Deep Creek Narrows. Looking up a tributary creek to the east, you can see the tangled jumble known as Devils Hole (not for hikers). Your trail swings northwest, passing above some sandy flats ideal for sunbathing, and intersects the steep jeep trail (3N34D) coming down from Bacon Flats 2.5 miles from the start. Leave the PCT here and descend the jeep trail 100 yards to Deep Creek. There is a large pool here deep enough for swimming.

Return the way you came. An option requiring a long car shuttle is to continue north and then northwest on the PCT to Deep Creek Hot Springs and then up to Bowen Ranch, 7 miles (see Hike 6).

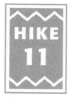

HOLCOMB CREEK

Hike Length: 12.75 miles one way; 2200' elevation gain
Difficulty: Strenuous (1 day), Moderate (2 days)
Season: April–October
Topo maps: *Lake Arrowhead , Butler Peak,* and *Fawnskin* (all 7.5')

Features

This is the longest hiking trip in the western half of the San Bernardinos. For 12.75 miles you follow the Pacific Crest Trail through silent forests of pine, cedar and oak, cross sparkling streams of cold water, and contour rocky slopes—quite an experience in this generally overused part of the range.

Most of the way you follow lower Holcomb Creek, either alongside the alder-shaded stream or a short distance above it. A third of the way, on a shady streamside bench, is Holcomb Crossing Trail Camp, the recommended overnight stop for those doing the trip in two days. A car shuttle between Hooks Creek Road and Coxey Road is required.

Here the 2003 Old Fire burned the forest 1.6 miles to the east of Deep Creek. This is an excellent opportunity for the hiker to view the fire devastation and to return in subsequent years to observe the regeneration of the forest. The steel bridge across Deep Creek was partially destroyed when a large burning pine tree crushed the east end of the bridge.

Description

From Highway 173 1.6 miles northeast of the junction with Highway 189 at Lake Arrowhead Village, drive east on Hook Creek Road through the village of Cedar Glen for 2.3 miles to a gate at Forest Service Road 2N26Y. Continue 0.8 mile down the windy one-lane road (with speed bumps!) and cross Little Bear Creek. Continue 0.1 mile on a good dirt road to a signed fork where 2N26Y meets a sharp bend in 3N34. Trail 3W12 from North Shore campground (Hike 9) ends close to this point. Stay left at the junction on 3N34. Cross the creek again and make a right turn at 3N34C after 0.2 mile. Pass another gate (**GPS SB10**) and proceed 0.3 mile to the Splinters Cabin Trailhead where the hike begins. If either gate is locked, park outside and walk from the gate, taking care not to block access to the gate or to private property on Hook Creek Road.

Arrange a second vehicle at the junction of Holcomb Creek and Coxey Road (2N14). To reach this junction from Fawnskin, turn northwest at the sign for Butler Peak onto Rim of the World Drive, which becomes 3N14. Follow it 4.4 miles from Fawnskin to the creek crossing and junction with 3N93 (**GPS SB11A**).

Take the distinct but unmarked trail down to Deep Creek, then go north along the west bank to a junction with the Pacific Crest Trail, 0.25 mile. At this point, the PCT crossed Deep Creek on a steel bridge. Until the bridge is repaired, follow detour markers. Do not attempt to wade the creek when the water is deep and fast, such as during storm conditions. After Deep Creek, your trail climbs eastward through chaparral, scrub oak, and scattered Jeffrey pines, with far-reaching views back over the Deep Creek drainage. In 2.5 miles you cross a ridge and begin a gentle descent into the Holcomb Creek watershed. You drop close to the creek, then contour about 100 feet above the south bank to a junction with the Crab Flats Trail (see Hike 14). About 300 yards beyond is Holcomb Crossing Trail Camp, on a Jeffrey-pine-shaded bench alongside the creek, with firepits and a toilet, 4.5 miles from the start.

Just east of the trail camp your trail makes a bouldery crossing of Holcomb Creek, then passes a junction with the Cox Creek Trail 2W03 (see Hike 18). You climb the slope to pass some rocky narrows, then descend back to Holcomb Creek at a cedar-shaded bench, 0.7 mile from the trail camp. Here you pass a junction with the Cienega Redonda Trail, branching northeast to Big Pine Flat. You continue east up Holcomb Creek, climb 100 feet on a chaparral slope, and then return to the creek to a junction with the Crab Flats Road (3N16) at **GPS SB11B**. This is an alternative endpoint if you prefer a shorter hike. Now you climb gradually eastward along the north slope above Holcomb Creek, through chaparral and open groves of ponderosa pine and oak, turn northeast, and finally drop back alongside the alder-shaded creek. Your trail continues northeast close to the creek, paralleling Forest Road 3N93 on the opposite bank. You pass several jeep tracks and reach a junction with Coxey Road (3N14). Here your transportation should be waiting. A longer option, recommended for 3 or 4 days, is to continue eastward on the Pacific Crest Trail to its crossing of either Van Dusen Road 3N09, (11 additional miles) or to Doble on the Gold Mountain Road 3N08 (17.5 additional miles).

HEAPS PEAK ARBORETUM

Hike Length: 0.7 mile round trip; 100' elevation gain
Difficulty: Easy
Season: April–November
Topo map: n/a

Features

The Heaps Peak Arboretum offers a pleasant stroll through trees and wild-flowers of the San Bernardino Mountains. It is built just above where Fred Heaps established a pioneering ranch in the late 1800s. The area burned in 1922 and was replanted by the Lake Arrowhead Women's Club with the assistance of students from the Lake Arrowhead Elementary School. The site was abandoned in the middle of the century but was restored in 1982 by George Hesemann and the Rim of the World Interpretive Association, which now maintains the arboretum.

The kiosk at the arboretum contains a display of the western pine bark beetle that has been decimating the forests of the San Bernardino Mountains. The beetle preys on trees weakened by the lengthy drought. It leaves forests of dead trees in its wake, tinder for the Old Fire and other fires yet to come.

Description

Park at a large turnout on the north side of Highway 18 (**GPS SB12**) two miles east of the Lake Arrowhead turnoff (Highway 173) and a quarter mile east of mile marker 27.00.

Pick up an interpretive trail guide at the Forest Information kiosk. The guide describes plants at twenty-five numbered posts along the loop. On weekends between 11:00 and 3:00, the Forest Information kiosk is staffed with volunteers when weather permits.

The Sequoia Trail is a 0.7 mile loop featuring a Sequoia grove, Arizona cypress, quaking aspen, California black oak, bracken fern, cinquefoil, rabbit brush, coffeeberry, potentilla, gooseberry, candytuft and any number of wildflowers. The loop is also a good place for bird watching. Portions of the arboretum were damaged by the Old Fire, but most of the trees are recovering.

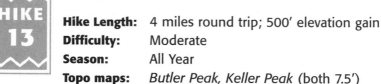

UPPER DEEP CREEK

Hike Length:	4 miles round trip; 500' elevation gain
Difficulty:	Moderate
Season:	All Year
Topo maps:	*Butler Peak, Keller Peak* (both 7.5')

Features

This trip drops from the rolling high country north of Green Valley into the upper reaches of Deep Creek. The trail is well maintained; the views are far-reaching; the forest is rich with Jeffrey and Coulter pines and several varieties of oak. Along Deep Creek is Fishermans Public Campground, popular with trout fisherman. Bring your fishing rod.

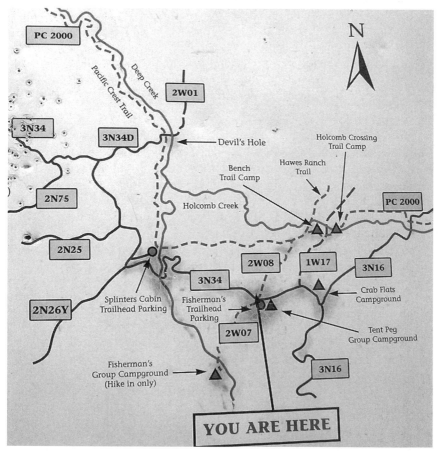

A helpful locator map of Deep Creek

Description

From the Rim of the World Highway (State Highway 18), 2.9 miles northeast of the intersection with 330 at Running Springs and just past mile marker 018 SBD 34.50, turn left (north) onto Green Valley Road. After 2.6 miles—just before you reach Green Valley Lake—turn left again onto Forest Road 3N16. Descend this good dirt road toward Crab Flats Campground, passing several side roads and crossing Crab Creek (impassible in high water). Reach the junction with Big Pine Flat Road after 3.8 miles. Stay left on 3N34, passing Crab Flats Campground after 0.2 mile. Another 1.1 miles farther, park at a clearing and large VISITORS TO DEEP CREEK sign near Tent Peg group camp (**GPS SB13**).

Follow trail 2W07 from the south side of the road as it contours west around a ridge, with fine views over the Deep Creek drainage and the north-slope country. After 0.25 mile the trail begins a descent into Deep Creek, crossing the small stream of Crab Creek after 1.5 miles, and reaching bottom at Fishermans Public Campground, 2 miles from the start.

After trying your luck as an angler, return back up the same way.

A winding dirt road comes down to Fishermans Camp from Cedar Glen, 8 miles west. This road is private property, owned by the Los Angeles Council of the Boy Scouts of America, and is closed to public travel. Hikers are allowed to use this road with permission, which allows for a superb shuttle overnight trip from Crab Flats to Cedar Glen. Contact the L. A. Area Council, 2333 Scout Way, Los Angeles, CA 90026.

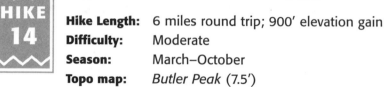

HOLCOMB CROSSING TRAIL CAMP

Hike Length: 6 miles round trip; 900′ elevation gain
Difficulty: Moderate
Season: March–October
Topo map: *Butler Peak* (7.5′)

Features

This is the easy way to reach the woodsy haunt of lower Holcomb Creek. You drop right down from Crab Flats to intersect the Pacific Crest Trail west of Holcomb Crossing Trail Camp.

The trip is a living demonstration of how the forest changes with access to moisture and heat. Most of the way down from Crab Flats you are in what botanists call Transition zone—Jeffrey pines, California black and canyon live oak, a scattering of Coulter and sugar pine and incense-cedar—trees that require a moderate amount of moisture and coolness. Directly across the canyon is Upper Sonoran vegetation, including pinyon pine and juniper trees that grow in warm, semi-arid conditions found on such south-facing slopes. And along Holcomb Creek are the lush trees of streamside wood-land—white alder, willow, and cottonwood—growing amid a verdant tangle of ferns, grasses and flowering herbs.

Description

From the Rim of the World Highway (State Highway 18), 2.9 miles north-east of the intersection with 330 at Running Springs and just past mile mark-er 018 SBD 34.50, turn left (north) onto Green Valley Road. After 2.6 miles—just before you reach Green Valley Lake—turn left again onto Forest Road 3N16. Descend this good dirt road toward Crab Flats Campground, passing several side roads and crossing Crab Creek (impassible in high water). Reach the junction with Big Pine Flat Road after 3.8 miles. Stay left on 3N34, passing Crab Flats Campground after 0.2 mile. Another 1.1 miles farther, park at a clearing and large VISITORS TO DEEP CREEK sign near Tent Peg group camp (**GPS SB13**).

The trail, 2W08, starts as an ATV track but soon narrows to a hiking trail. It gently climbs over a broad forested ridge, then drops northeastward into the Holcomb Creek Canyon, passing areas charred by fire. In 1.5 miles 2W08 ends at the Pacific Crest Trail. Turn right (east). In 0.5 miles, pass a signed junction with 2W03 leading north to Hawes Ranch. In 0.3 more miles, come to Bench Camp on a shady flat above the creek. In another 0.3 miles, pass an ATV track (1W17) climbing southward to Crab Flats. Shortly thereafter, arrive at Holcomb Crossing Trail Camp (**GPS SB14A**), located on a pine-canopied stream-side bench (fire pits and toilet).

You have several options on this trip: (1) return to Crab Flats the way you came; (2) climb the ATV track 1W17 steeply up 1.3 miles to Crab Flat (**GPS SB14B**), then walk west on 3N34 0.8 miles to the trailhead (3) follow the PCT west to Forest Road 3N34, then southeast back to Crab Flats; (4) follow the PCT east to Coxey Road (see Trip 11); or (5) follow the Cox Creek Trail north to Hawes Ranch (see Trip 18). The last two require a car shuttle. Any way you do it, you are certain to enjoy this bit of canyon wilderness smack in the middle of the overdeveloped western half of the San Bernardinos.

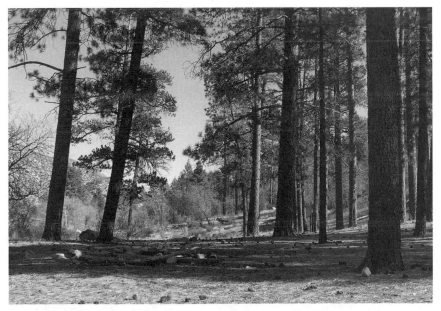

Holcomb Crossing Trail Camp

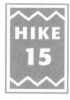

COXEY CREEK

Hike Length: 6 miles one way; 1400' elevation loss
Difficulty: Moderate
Season: November–May
Topo map: *Butler Peak, Lake Arrowhead, Keller Peak* (both 7.5')

Features

This trip crosses the pinyon-pine and juniper country of the semi-arid north side of the San Bernardinos. You descend westward along Coxey Creek (Mill Creek on topo map) for 3.5 miles, then cross open ridges for 2.5 miles down to Deep Creek. Although both the Forest Service map and the topographic map show a trail, actually you follow rough jeep tracks all the way. Do it in springtime, when Coxey Creek is running strong, and the aroma of damp sage and pinyon pine permeates the air. This hike follows an unmaintained and partially overgrown track. Long pants and gloves are recommended.

Description

From the Rim of the World Highway (State Highway 18), just past mile marker 018 SBD 34.50, turn left (north) onto Green Valley Road. After 2.6 miles—just before you reach Green Valley—turn left again onto Crab Flats Road (3N16). Descend 3N16 for 3.8 miles, passing several small side roads and crossing Crab Creek, to a signed junction with 3N34. Stay right on 3N16 and proceed for 8.3 more miles northeast to Big Pine Flat, watching the vegetation transition from forest to desert. Then turn left (west) on the Coxey Truck Trail (3N14) and follow it 4.6 miles to Coxey Meadow. Park in the clearing by the gate (**GPS SB15**).

Walk west along the jeep tracks that follow the north bank of Coxey Creek, usually alongside the stream, occasionally climbing to get past narrows. In 3.5 miles you pass Forest Road 3N59, cross Coxey Creek, and climb southward over a ridge. Another 0.5 mile and you begin the descent into the canyon of Deep Creek, 2 miles farther on.

You reach Deep Creek opposite the road down coming from Bacon Flats. Here, if you're doing the trip one way as recommended, your transportation should be waiting (see Hike 10 for driving directions to Deep Creek).

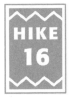

BARREL AND MUDDY SPRINGS

HIKE 16

Hike Length:	9 miles round trip; 1100' elevation gain
Difficulty:	Moderate
Season:	November–May
Topo map:	*Butler Peak, Keller Peak* (both 7.5')

Features

There are many running springs and water seepages in the San Bernardino Mountains, and most of them can be reached by road. This trip visits two little springs that can be reached only by walking. The springs themselves are not much to see, but the trail walk through stands of Jeffrey pine and pinyon, high on the ridgeside with sweeping views over lower Holcomb Creek and Deep Creek, is pleasant. From the high point of the trail you can see Lake Arrowhead sparkling in the distance. This is lonely mountain country, seldom visited except during hunting season; you should have the trail all to yourself. It is unmaintained and was badly burned during the 1999 Willow Fire. Nasty brush is growing back; long pants and gloves are recommended.

Description

From the Rim of the World Highway (State Highway 18), just past mile marker 018 SBD 34.50, turn left (north) onto Green Valley Road. After 2.6 miles—just before you reach Green Valley—turn left again onto Crab Flats Road (3N16). Descend 3N16 for 3.8 miles, passing several small side roads and crossing Crab Creek, to a signed junction with 3N34. Stay right on 3N16 and proceed for 8.3 more miles northeast to Big Pine Flat, watching the vegetation transition from forest to desert. Then turn left (west) on the Coxey Truck Trail (3N14) and follow it 3.4 miles to Little Pine Flat. Turn left on Hawes Ranch Road (3N41) and park in the clearing outside the locked gate (**GPS SB16**).

Hike past the gate and along 3N41 for 1.6 miles to its end just beyond the ranch. About 50 yards west of the HOLCOMB CREEK TRAIL sign (see Hike 18) is a wooden sign indicating MUDDY SPRING 3 MILES. Follow the trail—not a dirt road that soon ends—up the shallow gully westward, along a trickling creek, through a beautiful Jeffrey pine forest. In 1 mile you reach the saddle in the ridge between Little Shay and Shay mountains, from where Lake Arrowhead appears far to the southwest. The trail now drops down and follows the south slope of the ridge through pinyon pines. In 0.25 mile you come to the small seepage of Barrel Spring, just below the trail (water enough to drink during wet months). The trail then continues west, dropping 100' or more before climbing back up to the ridgetop, then descending northwest to Muddy Spring, overlooking Deep Creek basin, 1.25 miles from Barrel Spring. The water here also flows enough to use only during times of abundant rainfall. Return the same way.

SHAY MOUNTAIN

HIKE 17

Hike Length: 7 miles round trip; 1100' elevation gain
Difficulty: Moderate
Season: November–May
Topo map: *Butler Peak, Keller Peak* (both 7.5')

Features

The long hogback of Shay Mountain (6714') looms high over the north-side country of the San Bernardinos. From its broad summit one has panoramic views reaching from Lake Arrowhead almost to Big Bear and stretching far out over the Mojave Desert.

This trip is part on trail, part cross-country scramble. But the scrambling is easy climbing over pinyon-dotted slopes. Do it in spring, when the north-side country is damp and aromatic, and the high peaks to the southeast are glistening in their snowy mantle.

There have been lots of Shays in the history of the San Bernardinos. The particular Shay after whom the mountain is named is said to be an early-day ranger at the old Coxey Ranger Station, Art Shay.

This area was badly burned in the 1999 Willow Fire. Nasty brush is growing back. Cross-country navigation skills are essential.

Description

From the Rim of the World Highway (State Highway 18), just past mile marker 018 SBD 34.50, turn left (north) onto Green Valley Road. After 2.6 miles—just before you reach Green Valley—turn left again onto Crab Flats Road (3N16). Descend 3N16 for 3.8 miles, passing several small side roads and crossing Crab Creek, to a signed junction with 3N34. Stay right on 3N16 and proceed for 8.3 more miles northeast to Big Pine Flat, watching the vegetation transition from forest to desert. Then turn left (west) on the Coxey Truck Trail (3N14) and follow it 3.4 miles to Little Pine Flat. Turn left on Hawes Ranch Road (3N41) and park in the clearing outside the locked gate (**GPS SB16**).

Hike down the road to Hawes Ranch and proceed westward up the Muddy Spring Trail (see Hike 16) 1 mile to the ridgetop saddle. Then leave the trail and walk northwest along the upward slope, through open stands of pinyon pine, to the nearly-bare summit, 1 more mile. If you return to the trail saddle unfulfilled, scramble up the other direction (southeast) 0.75 mile to the top of Little Shay Mountain (6635').

COX CREEK

Hike Length: 6 miles round trip; 600' elevation gain
Difficulty: Moderate
Season: All year
Topo map: *Butler Peak, Keller Peak* (both 7.5')

Features

This is another route into the beautiful lower reaches of Holcomb Creek. You approach from the north, dropping down Cox Creek, then descending ridges and slopes into Holcomb Creek to Holcomb Crossing Trail Camp. Along Cox Creek are Jeffrey pines, but on the ridges and slopes you go through a semi-arid forest of pinyon pine and western juniper. In all but the hottest months, this is a very pleasant trail trip, with options when you reach Holcomb Crossing.

Description

From the Rim of the World Highway (State Highway 18), just past mile marker 018 SBD 34.50, turn left (north) onto Green Valley Road. After 2.6 miles—just before you reach Green Valley—turn left again onto Crab Flats Road (3N16). Descend 3N16 for 3.8 miles, passing several small side roads and crossing Crab Creek, to a signed junction with 3N34. Stay right on 3N16 and proceed for 8.3 more miles northeast to Big Pine Flat, watching the vegetation transition from forest to desert. Then turn left (west) on the Coxey Truck Trail (3N14) and follow it 3.4 miles to Little Pine Flat. Turn left on Hawes Ranch Road (3N41) and park in the clearing outside the locked gate (**GPS SB16**).

Hike down the road for 1.6 miles to Hawes Ranch. A wooden sign pointing south along Cox Creek indicates HOLCOMB CREEK 3 MILES. For 1 mile the trail follows the creek, through a magnificent forest of Jeffrey pine. The trail climbs to near the top of the ridge immediately east of the creek and follows this pinyon-covered ridge down to a little open valley on the north side of Holcomb Creek. On the north bank of the creek you intersect the Pacific Crest Trail (see Hike 11). Turn right (west), cross the creek via boulders, and in 100 yards reach shady Holcomb Crossing Trail Camp.

You can return the way you came or, with a car shuttle, take the Pacific Crest Trail in either direction (see Hike 11), or, 300 yards west of the trail camp, find the trail that heads southwest to Crab Flats (see Hike 14).

EXPLORATION TRAIL

HIKE
19

Hike Length: 4 miles one way; 1300' elevation gain
Difficulty: Moderate
Season: April–November
Topo map: *Keller Peak* (7.5')

Features

The Exploration Trail was completed in August 2005 as part of the Forest Service Centennial Project to celebrate the 100th birthday of the U.S. Forest Service. It parallels the Keller Peak road through beautiful open oak and pine forest to the top of the road where it meets the National Children's Forest Interpretive Trail. For an easier trip, follow the trail in reverse, downhill all the way.

While you are in the area, consider walking the short Interpretive Trail and visiting the historic Keller Peak Fire Lookout.

Description

From Highway 18 at a bend just east of Running Springs at mile marker 18 SBD 32.81, turn right (east) on the paved Keller Peak road and drive 0.1 mile. Park at the signed Exploration Trail trailhead on the right (**GPS SB19**). Leave another car or bicycle at the upper end of the trail, 4 miles up the paved Keller Peak Road (**GPS SB19A**). The trailhead is on the right side just beyond a fork in the road; the left fork leads to the National Children's Forest Interpretive Trail.

Two trails depart from the lower trailhead; take the one on the right. The trail crosses Dry Creek, then climbs alongside it through an open forest of oak and pine past huge granite boulders for half a mile to a dirt road. Cross the road, then hike another quarter mile and cross a second road.

From here, the trail continues climbing, roughly parallel to the Keller Peak Road. It passes through fields of chaparral, then returns to open forest and contours across the northwest slopes of Keller Peak to its upper terminus at the paved road.

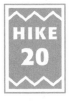

LITTLE GREEN VALLEY

Hike Length: 3 miles one way; 700' elevation gain
Difficulty: Moderate
Season: April–November
Topo map: *Keller Peak* (7.5')

Features

Before the loggers and subdividers arrived on the scene, the top of the San Bernardinos from Crestline to Big Bear was heavily clothed in tall timber. Today, stands of magnificent pine, cedar, and oak, undisturbed by humans, are rare and widely scattered. One place where you can still find them, rich and tall and verdant, is on the ridges north of Snow Valley. This is a beautiful walk through the realm of these forest monarchs, on good trail or fire road all the way, and sometimes beside a trickling stream. Do it on a day when you have plenty of time, so that you can saunter, pause, and fully soak up nature's handiwork. The trip is especially pleasant in the spring when the creek is running and in the autumn when the oak leaves are turning yellow.

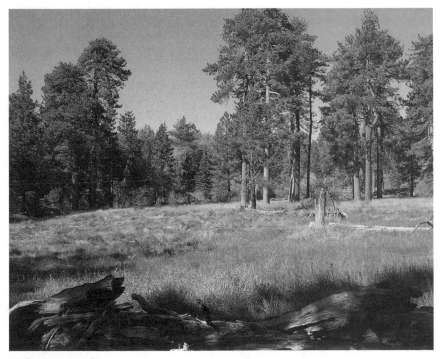

Little Green Valley

Description

Drive up the Rim of the World Highway (State Highway 18) to mile marker 038 SBD 37.24, 0.3 mile west of the Snow Valley parking area and 5 miles east of Running Springs. A dirt road forks left (north) to some cabins; turn off the highway, then turn left immediately again and park in the clearing on the left where you see the 2W10 GREEN VALLEY TRAIL sign (**GPS SB20**).

You may wish to leave a second vehicle in Green Valley. From Highway 38 just east of mile marker 018 SBD 34.50, turn north on Green Valley Road and follow it 4.1 miles to Meadow Lane. Make a right and drive 0.3 miles to the unmarked dirt road 2N19 where Meadow Lane makes a sharp turn just beneath a water tank (**GPS SB20A**).

Follow the trail as it leads northwest, crosses a small brook, and gently climbs the slope. You cross two logging roads during the first 0.5 mile, the result of recent selective tree-cutting. After another 0.3 miles, stay left at an unmarked fork and climb the forested ridge to reach Little Green Valley. This is a good turnaround point if you want a short scenic walk without a car shuttle.

The trail briefly becomes indistinct as it traverses the south side of the marshy meadow and crosses a creek. Here you reach a dirt road 2N19 leading northwest to Green Valley Lake. Ignoring several forks, follow the dirt road across a ridge and down into the basin of Green Valley Lake. Pass just behind the Green Valley Public Campground, to Meadow Lane, 3 miles from the start.

If you have employed a car shuttle, your trip is over. Otherwise return the way you came.

SIBERIA CREEK TRAIL CAMP FROM SNOW VALLEY

Hike Length: 8.5 miles round trip; 2000′ elevation gain
Difficulty: Moderate
Season: All year
Topo map: *Keller Peak* (7.5′)

Features

A major fire raged through the Bear Creek drainage in 1971. Since then, the chaparral cover on the mountain slopes has grown back as vigorous as ever. The fire spared most of the canyon bottom and its lush streamside growth. Here, bigcone Douglas-fir, white alder, and canyon live oak protect the bubbling creek and its grassy banks from the sun's harshness.

Merging with Bear Creek just across from where the trail reaches canyon bottom is beautiful, woodsy Siberia Creek, probably the most delightful sylvan recess in the San Bernardinos outside of the San Gorgonio Wilderness.

Its little singing stream, shaded by an over-arching canopy of green, is a favorite of hikers, campers and fishermen alike. Here, smack in the middle of the overused San Bernardinos, nature reveals her quiet, pristine best.

This trip leaves the Rim of the World Highway (State Highway 18), drops down chaparral-clad slopes into Bear Creek, then continues into the deep, verdant oasis of Siberia Creek—miraculously untouched by the holocaust that ravaged the slopes just above. Here, just above the junction with Bear Creek, the Forest Service has placed Siberia Creek Trail Camp—stoves, tables, and toilet. Bring your fishing rod; rainbow trout swim in nearby Bear Creek.

At the time of this writing, the trail is very brushy. The Forest Service hopes to send in a trail crew in Spring 2006; contact the Big Bear Discovery Center for up-to-date conditions.

Description

Drive 5.5 miles east of Running Springs (0.5 mile past Snow Valley) on State Highway 18 to mile marker 18 SBD 38.00. Turn right onto the poor dirt Forest Service road 2N97. Low clearance vehicles may wish to park near the highway. Otherwise, drive up the deeply rutted road, staying left at a fork, to a small parking area on the right on a ridgetop, 0.4 mile from the highway (**GPS SB21**). A sign here for the Camp Creek Trail (1W09) reads BEAR CREEK.

Take the trail eastward, over the ridge, under scattered Jeffrey pines. In 0.5 mile you reach the 1971 burn, and the forest changes to chaparral, with a few blackened stumps jutting skyward. The trail now zigzags steeply down the brushy slopes to the welcome shade and cool water of Bear Creek, 4 miles. You cross Bear Creek, enter the mouth of Siberia Creek, and reach

Siberia Creek Trail Camp, located on an alder- and oak-shaded bench just north of the stream.

Return the same way. Or, with car shuttle, take the trail northeast into the Bluff Lake country (see Hike 30), or the trail south to Seven Pines (see Hike 39).

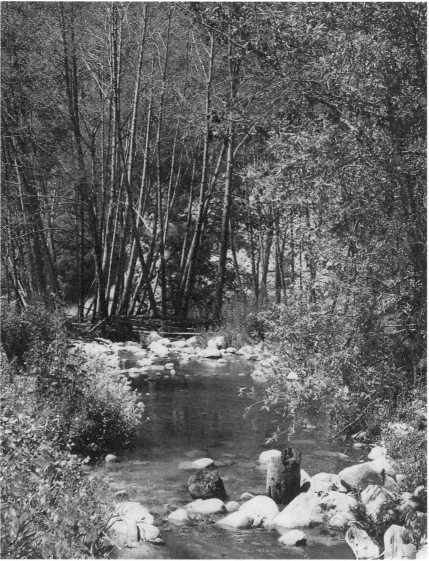

Siberia Creek

John W. Robinson

GRAYS PEAK

Hike Length: 6 miles round trip; 1200' elevation gain
Difficulty: Moderate
Season: April–October
Topo map: *Fawnskin* (7.5')

Features

Forested 7952-foot Grays Peak looms close over the western end of Big Bear Lake. The peak is named for Gray's Landing on the north shore of the lake, founded by Alex Gray in 1918 and still used by anglers.

This is an easy-graded, very pleasant walk through stands of Jeffrey pine, black oak, and white fir, partly on a newly constructed trail, partly on fire road. The trailhead is in the center of a bald eagle wintering habitat area and is closed to public use from November 1 to April 1.

Description

Follow State Highway 38 along the north shore of Big Bear Lake to the Grays Peak parking area (**GPS SB22**) just west of mile marker 038 SBD 56.41, 2.7 miles northeast of Big Bear Dam, or half a mile southwest of Fawnskin. There are restrooms and picnic tables here, and many spaces for parking.

The signed trailhead is at the north edge of the picnic-parking area. Follow the pathway as it gently climbs through open forest to intersect a dirt fire road 2N04X, 0.5 mile. Turn right onto the road, going straight ahead at a road junction with 2N70, to a signed junction with the Grays Peak Trail, another 0.5 mile. Turn left and follow the trail as it climbs, contours, and climbs again, circling around to the south flank of the peak. The trail ends 100 feet below the top; work your way through buckthorn thickets and downed trees to the summit. Views are limited by the forest cover, but you can make out shimmering Big Bear Lake to the south, and the rugged lower Holcomb Creek country to the north.

Return the way you came.

DELAMAR MOUNTAIN

HIKE 23

Hike Length: 5 miles round trip; 1000' elevation gain
Difficulty: Moderate
Season: April–November
Topo map: *Fawnskin* (7.5')

Features

Delamar Mountain stands 8398' tall on the divide separating the Holcomb Creek drainage from Big Bear Lake. From its rocky, forested summit, you are rewarded with a superb panorama of the central San Bernardinos, with sparkling-blue Big Bear Lake immediately to the south and Holcomb Valley's historic gold country right below to the north.

This trip follows a fairly new stretch of the Pacific Crest Trail for two miles, then climbs the east ridge of Delamar Mountain through an open forest of Jeffrey pine and white fir. Since part of it is trailless, wear boots with deep tread.

Description

From State Highway 38, 2 miles east of Fawnskin at mile marker 038 SBD 54.04, turn north onto the good dirt Polique Canyon Road (2N09). At a fork in 1.5 miles with 2N71, stay right on 2N09 toward Holcomb Valley. Continue 0.8 mile to the top of the divide, where you will see the signed Holcomb View Trail, part of the Pacific Crest Trail (**GPS SB23**). Park here or on the side of the road where it becomes wider just beyond.

Walk west on the Pacific Crest Trail, ascending gradually along the south side of the Big Bear-Holcomb Valley divide. You pass through an open forest of conifer and oak, with numerous views south to Big Bear Lake. In 1.5 miles you cross to the shadier north slope of the ridge and then contour northwest another 0.5 mile. At the point where the PCT begins a steady descent, leave the trail and climb westward on an easy cross-country ascent to Delamar Mountain's forested east ridge. In 0.5 mile of trailless walking you reach the pile of rocks that is the summit (8398'). For the best view southward over Big Bear Lake, scramble about 100 yards south to a slightly lower summit.

Return the same way, or continue westward on the PCT to Delamar Mountain Road, Forest Road 3N12, which you reach at a point 3.5 miles north of Fawnskin. A car shuttle is required for this option.

BERTHA PEAK

Hike Length: 7 miles round trip; 1400' elevation gain
Difficulty: Moderate
Season: April–November
Topo map: *Fawnskin* (7.5')

Features

Like neighboring Delamar Mountain, Bertha Peak at 8201 feet rises high on the forested ridge between Holcomb Valley and Big Bear Lake. From its rounded summit, you get a striking perspective over the gentle valley-and-ridge country of the central San Bernardinos.

This trip takes the Cougar Crest Trail from State Highway 38, on the north shore of Big Bear Lake, to the Pacific Crest Trail, then ascends a steep dirt track to the electronic relay station on the summit. It is a pleasant and popular walk through an open forest of pinyon pine and juniper, climaxed by a panoramic view well worth the effort. Do it on a clear day, when almost the entire San Bernardinos sprawl below you, and the great Greyback–Mt. San Bernardino ridge looms high and stark on the southeast skyline.

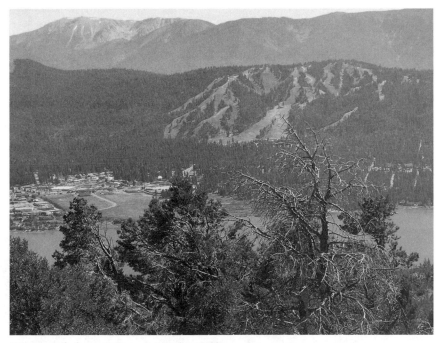

View south from PCT near Bertha Peak

Description

From Fawnskin, drive east on State Highway 38 2.5 miles to a large paved parking area on the north side of the highway near mile marker 038 SBD 53.50 with the sign COUGAR CREST TRAIL (**GPS SB24**). (If you reach the Big Bear Discovery Center, you've driven 0.2 mile too far.) Park here.

Walk up the well-marked Cougar Crest Trail (1E22), through an open forest of pinyon pine, juniper, and scattered Jeffrey pines as you wind upward toward Bertha Peak's west ridge. Panoramic views open over the Big Bear Lake country as you gain elevation, and in 2.3 miles you intersect the PCT. This is a popular turnaround point for families with young hikers. Turn right (east) and follow the PCT to a junction with a dirt road on the ridge crest, 0.5 mile. Walk up this dirt road, very steep in places, through pinyon pines and some rather large western junipers, to the summit relay station (**GPS SB24A**).

After taking in the 360-degree panorama, return the way you came.

GOLD MOUNTAIN

Hike Length: 4 miles round trip; 1000' elevation gain
Difficulty: Moderate
Season: April–November
Topo map: *Big Bear City* (7.5')

Features

The eastern and northern flanks of the San Bernardino Mountains are honeycombed with abandoned gold prospects. No other mountain region in Southern California has seen so much mining excitement spread over so many years—from the 1850s well into this century.

Of all the lode-mining operations in the range, none was as storied nor as famous as Lucky Baldwin's Gold Mountain (or Doble) Mine high on the mountainside overlooking Baldwin Lake. The rich quartz ledges were discovered in 1873 by prospectors Barney and Charley Carter. Their discovery turned out to be a mountain of gold ore, and the rush was on. Elias J. "Lucky" Baldwin bought "Carter's Quartz Hill" for $6,000,000, and by 1875 he had constructed a 40-stamp mill to process the ore and employed 180 men. Baldwin was not as "lucky" in this venture as he was in others, and it is doubtful that he ever saw a full return on his investment. During the early 1900s the mine was worked by several lessees, the most recent operation being in the late 1940s. The end finally came in 1951, when the equipment was removed and the property abandoned.

The site of the large mill and cyanide-processing plant can still be seen on the northeast slopes of Gold Mountain. This trip visits these storied ruins and climbs the pinyon-covered ridge of Gold Mountain for a panoramic view encompassing most of the old mining areas. For those with vivid imaginations, it is possible to look down over Doble Mine, Holcomb Valley, Arrastre Flat, and Van Dusen Canyon and visualize the feverish excitement and hectic activity that once occurred here. This trip is for those with such imaginations.

Description

From State Highway 18 at mile marker 018 SBD 58.15 where it makes its loop around the north end of Baldwin Lake, turn left (north) onto Holcomb Valley Road. Drive up this paved road 0.9 mile. Just before the dump, turn left on the dirt road 3N16. After 0.8 mile, stay left on 3N16 at a junction. Climb 0.1 more miles and park in the clearing across from the old wooden "hopper." (**GPS SB25**)

Before starting out on foot, look south along the mountainside, toward Baldwin Lake; the foundations and diggings you see are all that remain of this most famous lode mine in the San Bernardinos.

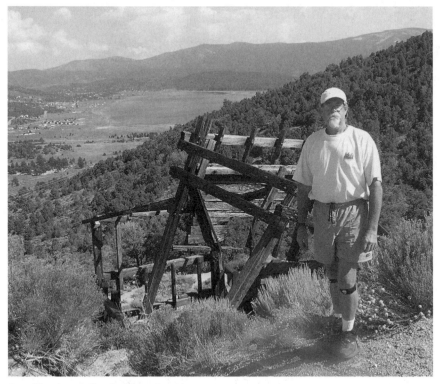

Joe Sheehy at the Doble mine

Walk up the dirt road about 200 yards, then start up the gentle, pinyon- and juniper-covered northeast ridge of Gold Mountain. The climb is trailless but easy going. Proceed around the right (north) side of a false summit to a junction with the Pacific Crest Trail, 1 mile. Continue up the broad pinyon-clad ridge to the 8235-foot summit of Gold Mountain for far-reaching views over this mine-poxed northeastern corner of the San Bernardinos.

Return the same way. An attractive option requiring a short car or bicycle shuttle (1.25 miles) is to descend via the PCT. You will get a good panorama of Baldwin Lake's usually dry playa where Budd Doble, Lucky Baldwin's son-in-law, once trained race horses. The PCT reaches Holcomb Valley Road 0.1 mile south of the dump (**GPS SB25A**).

SILVER PEAK

Hike Length: 4 miles round trip; 1000' elevation gain
Difficulty: Moderate
Season: All year
Topo map: *Big Bear City* (7.5')

Features

The desert-tempered north slope of the San Bernardinos holds delightful surprises. When winter's snowy mantle grips the higher parts of the range, this land of pinyon, juniper, and Joshua trees is warm and inviting. This trip samples this semi-arid terrain. You climb the grayish hogback of Silver Peak—partly on old mining roads, partly by cross-country scrambling—for a far-reaching view over the Mojave Desert and its islands of treeless, steep-sided tawny mountain ranges.

Blackhawk Mountain (the summit of which is called Silver Peak) was once the scene of gold and silver mining activities. Abandoned diggings and shafts dot the slopes on all sides. The greatest activity was in Blackhawk Canyon, down the north side of the mountain. Gold deposits were discovered here in 1887 and developed soon afterward by the Blackhawk Mining Company, financed by English capital. Tunnels were dug and a 10-stamp mill erected, but high operating costs forced suspension of the venture within a few years. In 1921 the mines were reopened by the Arlington Mining Corporation, and they were worked continuously until 1940, yielding a reported $300,000. Since 1940 they have been idle.

Cactus Flat, where the hike begins, commemorates "Cactus Jim" Johnson, builder of the Johnson Grade road up Cushenbury Canyon to Baldwin Lake. Old Cactus Jim selected his own burial site here, where his grave is now located and marked with a small sign.

Description

From the north shore of Big Bear Lake, proceed east on State Highway 18. Low-clearance vehicles may park at mile marker 62.0 and call box 18-618 (**GPS SB26A**). Otherwise, turn east onto a poor dirt road. Follow this side road 0.3 miles to the first dirt road on the left; turn left and continue 0.2 miles to a small parking area before the road drops down a hill and deteriorates badly. Park here (**GPS SB26**). Look north toward prominent white mine tailings at the toe of a ridge. Your route ascends the canyon behind these tailings, then follows the skyline to the summit.

Follow this dirt road 0.1 mile down into a gully, then turn left and hike up the gully 0.2 mile more to its end at another dirt road (a maze of old mining roads crisscross the mountain). Proceed right and follow this dirt road to the abandoned mine. Switchback northward through the white rock to

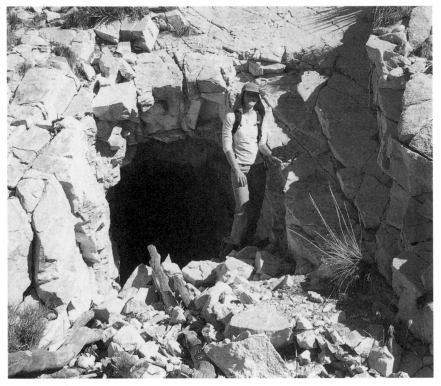

Mine on Silver Peak

the end of the path at an old mine shaft in the canyon. Turn up the canyon, roughly following a cable, to its top on the ridgeline. Climb up the spur ridge to the main ridge, where you will intersect another dirt road. Turn right (east) and follow the road up the main ridge to the 6756-foot summit (**GPS SB26B**).

Return the same way, avoiding the private property area on the southwest flank of the mountain, where exploratory mining work is being done.

CHAMPION JOSHUA TREE

Hike Length: 1 mile round trip; 100' elevation gain
Difficulty: Easy
Season: October–May
Topo map: *Big Bear City, Rattle Snake Canyon* (both 7.5')

Features

In the broad, desert-draining canyon of Arrastre Creek and its east fork, on the north slope of the San Bernardinos, was one of the most magnificent Joshua tree forests in the world. The shaggy Joshua tree is the oddest of all plants in these mountains. This weird giant of the lily family has bayonet-like leaves and a trunk with no annual rings and, therefore, no way to tell how old it is. In the springtime, clusters of greenish white, bell-shaped flowers with a rather unpleasant odor appear. Native Americans relished the roasted flower buds, and obtained a dye from the tree's red roots. Mormon settlers gave the tree its name; they saw a likeness to Joshua praying in the wilderness with his arms uplifted to the heavens. The tree owes its continued existence to the little Pronuba moth. The Joshua relies on the moth for pollination, and the moth larvae rely on the Joshua for food. Each depends on the other for its survival.

The largest Joshua tree in the world—discovered in 1967 and named "The Champion"—grew here at the foot of Granite Peak. This overgrown, shaggy monarch of the high desert was 14' 11" in circumference and over 32' high. A jeep track used to lead to the base of the tree, which was a popular site for Bacchanalian revelry. The Champion toppled over recently, killed by hooligans firing their guns into its trunk. This trip is a short stroll through a forest of pinyon pine, western juniper, and Joshua trees to the Champion. The jeep trail has been closed to reduce the impact on the area and threat to remaining large Joshua trees.

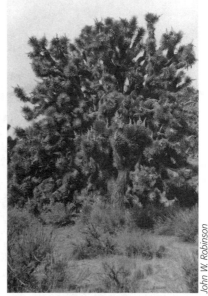

The Champion, once the largest known Joshua tree in the world

Description

Drive 3.5 miles northeast of Baldwin Lake on State Highway 18. At the sign pointing to Cactus Flats just past mile marker 18 SBD 61.00, turn right (southeast) onto Forest Road 3N03, Smarts Ranch Road (good dirt), and follow it 4.9 miles up the valley of Arrastre Creek to the creek crossing. Low clearance vehicles may wish to park on the right here (**GPS SB27A**), depending on the condition of hill beyond the creek. High clearance vehicles can continue 0.2 mile, then turn left and drive 0.3 mile to a large fenced parking area (**GPS SB27B**).

Look east-northeast toward Granite Peak and identify the grove of Joshua trees at the base. Your goal is to reach this grove. The path starts through a gap in the fence on the east side of the parking area. It follows a partially overgrown trail, then the faint old jeep tracks. Follow the track for a half mile to the big trees. On your right as you enter the grove, you'll see the fallen remains of the Champion, which once dwarfed the other large Joshuas around it.

The tracks turn south and follow the base of the rocky slopes past more Joshua trees. Explore the area, taking care not to stick yourself on any of the wickedly barbed cholla cactus.

Return the way you came.

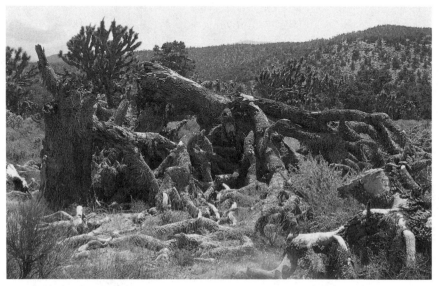

Dead Champion Tree

CASTLE ROCK

HIKE 28

Hike Length:	2 miles round trip; 700' elevation gain
Difficulty:	Moderate
Season:	April–October
Topo map:	*Big Bear Lake* (7.5')

Features

South from Big Bear Lake, rising from the heavily forested ridge that divides the Big Bear basin from the canyon of the Santa Ana River, are a number of granite knobs and boulder outcroppings. Most impressive of these is a weather-eroded, knobby gendarme known as Castle Rock.

Castle Rock has long attracted attention because of its sentrylike position above the lower end of the lake and its unusual shape. Such qualities impress human imaginations, and from these imaginations legends arise that persist through the ages. The legend of Castle Rock is one of the most famous of those known to Native Americans who once made the San Bernardinos their home.

This trip climbs steeply up the forested mountainside. You follow a trail to the foot of the rock; then it is a Class 3 scramble to the summit. Wear boots with good tread. Do it when a breeze freshens the mountains; perhaps you will be able to hear the soft wail of the forlorn Native American princess who waited for her husband on Castle Rock.

Description

From State Highway 18 across from mile marker 018 SBD 45.50, 1.2 mile east of Big Bear Dam or 3 miles west of Big Bear Lake Village, the marked trail 1W03 starts up a forested gully. Park 100 yards east of the trailhead in a clearing on the north side of the highway (**GPS SB28**).

The trail climbs steeply up the left (east) side of the gully through a magnificent forest of ponderosa pine, white fir and incense-cedar, passing jumbo granite boulders. In about 0.25 mile the trail reaches a saddle and starts to descend. Castle Rock is the large outcropping immediately east of this saddle. Leave the trail here. The easiest way up the rock (Class 3) is to contour about 50 feet around the north and west sides of the outcropping, then climb up an indentation to the summit. There is one spot about half way up where a belay may be warranted for the unsteady.

Descend the same way. Or with a prepositioned vehicle, hike south to Forest Service Road 2N86.

CHAMPION LODGEPOLE PINE

HIKE
29

Hike Length: 1 mile round trip; 50′ elevation gain
Difficulty: Easy
Season: April–October
Topo map: *Big Bear Lake* (7.5′)

Features

Lodgepole pines seldom grow taller than 70 feet, and in Southern California they are seldom seen below 8000 feet. An exception to these rules occurs in the vicinity of Bluff Lake, a shallow body of water surrounded by lush forest and meadow country, 3 miles south of Big Bear Lake. Here, at 7500′, grow the largest lodgepole pines in the world. The world champion, discovered in 1963, is a mammoth, double-topped tree standing 110′ tall with a circumference of 20′. Its age is estimated at 400 years, meaning that the tree's life has spanned California's history since shortly after Juan Rodriguez Cabrillo's epic voyage into San Diego Bay in 1542.

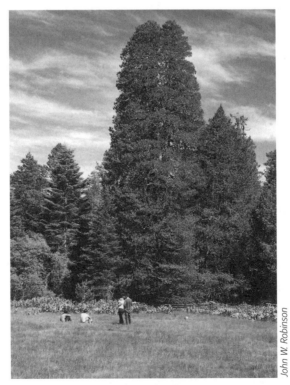

World Champion Lodgepole pine

Lodgepole—also known as tamarack—pines are readily identified by their thin, scaly bark and their paired needles (the only pine in these mountains with two needles per bundle). They are usually found only in high subalpine forests, just below timberline. This trip is a very short stroll through lush forest and grassland to the world champion. The trail is marked with several numbered posts. A pamphlet at the trailhead explains the sights at each post.

Description
From the west end of Big Bear Lake Village at mile marker 018 SBD 47.45 at a sign pointing to Mill Creek Road and picnic grounds, turn south onto Tulip Lane. Proceed 0.4 mile, then turn right on Mill Creek Road, which becomes good dirt Forest Service Road 2N10 in 0.7 mile. Proceed 3.8 miles, then turn right on 2N11 at a sign pointing to Champion Lodgepole. Proceed 1.0 miles to a signed parking area on the right for the 1W11 Lodgepole Pine Trail (**GPS SB29**).

Follow the trail west 0.3 mile alongside a trickling stream to a junction with 1W04 dropping to Siberia Creek. Then go right (north) 100 yards to Champion Lodgepole, near the east end of a meadow. Stay outside the wooden fence built by the Forest Service to protect the tree.

Return the same way.

SIBERIA CREEK

HIKE 30

Hike Length:	13 miles round trip; 2500' elevation gain
Difficulty:	Strenuous
Season:	April–October
Topo maps:	*Big Bear Lake, Keller Peak* (both 7.5')

Features

Siberia Creek begins in the shallow pond known as Bluff Lake, on the high tableland between Big Bear Lake and the valley of the Santa Ana River. It flows southwest across this lushly forested tableland, through magnificent stands of white fir, ponderosa and lodgepole pine, and emerald-green meadows of tall grass, ferns, and flowering herbs. Then it abruptly drops down a boulder-filled gorge, finally to empty its spent waters into Bear Creek. Here, set amid alders, oaks and spruces, is Siberia Creek Trail Camp (stoves, tables and toilet).

A trail descends most of the length of Siberia Creek—from the west end of Forest Road 2N11 two miles south of Bluff Lake all the way down to Siberia Creek Trail Camp, where it joins the trail up to the Rim of the World Highway (State Highway 18) (see Hike 21). This trip follows this trail—first across the verdant tableland, then down around the steep slopes of Lookout Point to avoid the difficult gorge, and into lower Siberia Creek and its small trail camp. From here, options are available with a car shuttle (see below).

The trail is badly overgrown and presently requires crawling through brush in places. The Forest Service hopes to send in a trail crew in Spring 2006; contact the Big Bear Discovery Center for up-to-date conditions.

Description

From the west end of Big Bear Lake Village at mile marker 018 SBD 47.45 at a sign pointing to Mill Creek Road and picnic grounds, turn south onto Tulip Lane. Proceed 0.4 mile, then turn right on Mill Creek Road, which becomes good dirt Forest Service Road 2N10 in 0.7 mile. Proceed 3.8 miles, then turn right on 2N11 at a sign pointing to Champion Lodgepole. Proceed 1 mile to a signed parking area on the right for the 1W11 Lodgepole Pine Trail (**GPS SB29**).

From the parking area on Forest Road 2N11, follow the Lodgepole Pine Trail 0.3 mile west, alongside a small creek, to a fork. Consider taking the 100 yard excursion to the right to see the Champion Lodgepole tree (see Hike 29). Otherwise, continue straight ahead on 1W04, alongside lush meadowland and through open forest. In 0.75 mile you cross Siberia Creek and follow its north bank downstream; 0.25 mile farther you recross the creek. Here the tableland ends and the stream abruptly drops into a boulder-stacked gorge. Follow the trail as it contours out onto the open-forested slopes of Lookout Mountain, drops to a saddle, and zigzags down the steep ridge westward to a junction with the Seven Pines Trail (see Hike 39), 5 miles from the start. Turn right (north) and follow the latter one mile down to Siberia Creek Trail Camp, located alongside the stream to your left, just before Siberia Creek meets Bear Creek.

Return the same way, all uphill now. Or, with a car shuttle, ascend the Green Valley Trail to the Rim of the World Highway (State Highway 18) (see Hike 21) or the Seven Pines Trail to Seven Pines (see Hike 39). Any way you do it, consider spending the night at Siberia Creek Trail Camp.

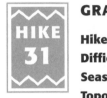

GRAND VIEW POINT

Hike Length: 6 miles round trip; 1200′ elevation gain
Difficulty: Moderate
Season: May–October
Topo map: *Big Bear Lake* (7.5′)

Features
This trip climbs from the new Aspen Glen Picnic Ground to the summit of the high ridge that separates Bear Valley from the basin of the Santa Ana River. En route you are rewarded with occasional views over Big Bear Lake and its crowded resort complex, and from aptly named Grand View Point you look across the deep trench of the Santa Ana to the lofty peaks and ridges of the San Gorgonio Wilderness. You're on trail or fire road all the way to Grand View Point. On weekends this trail is popular with horseback riders.

Description
From the west end of Big Bear Lake Village at mile marker 018 SBD 47.45 at a sign pointing to Mill Creek Road and picnic grounds, turn south onto Tulip Lane. Proceed 0.4 mile, then stay left and continue 0.1 more miles to the Aspen Glen picnic area on your right (**GPS SB31**).

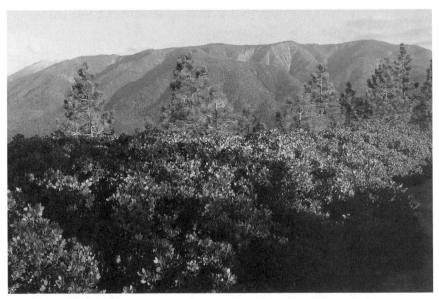

San Bernardino Ridge from near Grand View Point

The Pineknot Trail, 1E01, starts at the extreme east end of the parking area, just above the road. In 50 yards go left at a fork and follow the trail over a rise and down into a willow-choked draw. Turn right at a second trail junction and follow the broad path as it ascends the draw, then climbs above it, under a shady canopy of Jeffrey pine, black oak, and white fir. You climb to a spur road (2N93Y), then follow this road up to a junction with Forest Road 2N10 at the top of the ridge. Cross the road and follow the marked trail 0.25 mile southeast to the open summit of Grand View Point for a panorama of the eastern San Bernardinos that is truly grand.

Return the same way, or cut the trip in half by having transportation awaiting you on Forest Road 2N10.

SUGARLOAF MOUNTAIN FROM GREEN CANYON

Hike Length: 10 miles round trip; 2000' elevation gain
Difficulty: Moderate
Season: May–October
Topo map: *Moonridge* (7.5')

Features

Sugarloaf Mountain—as the name implies—is a massive rounded lump on the main divide between the Big Bear country and the canyon of the Santa Ana River. From its 9952' forested summit, you are treated to an all-encompassing vista over the whole eastern half of the San Bernardinos. It is the highest peak in the range outside of the San Gorgonio Wilderness.

For a mountain almost 10,000 feet high, Sugarloaf displays a surprising variety of flora. The usual Jeffrey pine, sugar pine, white fir, and incensecedar are found along the summit ridge and in sheltered recesses. Near the summit are some teepee-like western junipers. Pinyon pine, juniper, and mountain mahogany abound on the middle slopes, and purple sage and skeleton weed are prevalent in the sparsely forested sections. The rare black swallowtail butterfly, *Papilio bairdi*, can be seen on the summit in late August and early September.

This trail trip ascends beautifully forested Green Canyon to the top of the ridge, then follows the ridge westward to the summit. It is an ideal jaunt for a warm summer day, when the cool breezes along the ridgetop offer refreshing relief from the sweltering valley below.

Description

Drive east, then south on State Highway 38 from Big Bear City. About 3 miles from town, turn right onto the good dirt Forest Road 2N93. The turnoff is across from Hatchery Road near the 038 SBD 45.75 mile marker. Follow 2N93, passing several small side roads, as it curves left and climbs along the mountainside to the Green Creek crossing. Park at the signed Sugarloaf Trail 2E18 (**GPS SB32**), 1.3 miles from State Highway 38.

Walk up the steep dirt road that turns to jeep tracks in a short distance, following alongside trickling Green Creek. When you reach the saddle atop the ridge and a trail junction, turn right (west) and follow the ridgetop trail 2E02 to the forested summit.

Return the same way. An option, requiring a car shuttle, is to descend to the saddle junction, then join Hikes 33 or 34.

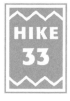

SUGARLOAF MOUNTAIN
FROM WILDHORSE MEADOWS

Hike Length: 7 miles roundtrip; 1300' elevation gain
Difficulty: Moderate
Season: May–October
Topo map: *Moonridge* (7.5')

Features

This is the shortest and easiest way to climb Sugarloaf Mountain, but it involves a drive over a narrow and in some places rocky dirt road. You climb from Wildhorse Meadows up to the saddle east of Sugarloaf, then follow the ridgetop to the summit, on trail all the way. (For more on Sugarloaf Mountain, see Hike 32.)

Description

From Redlands drive east on State Highway 38 through Barton Flats to the beginning of Forest Road 2N93 near mileage marker 038 SBD 35.7 (**GPS SB33A**). The fair dirt road is easy to pass by, so keep a sharp eye out for it on your left (north) immediately past a small wash. Drive up Forest Road 2N93

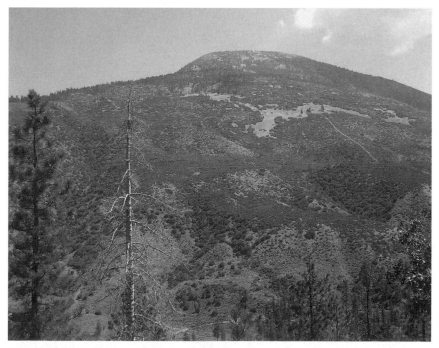

Sugarloaf Mountain from the southwest

to Wildhorse Meadows, 5.5 miles. Continue up 2N93 0.6 mile beyond the meadow, to a fork on your left with a steep jeep road (easy to miss). Park here (**GPS SB33**); there is a locked gate blocking the jeep road.

Pass through a wooden break in the fence and walk west, following ducks up another jeep road, to the top of the ridge. Here the road divides into several indistinct jeep paths. Continue west, atop the ridge, then drop to a 4-way trail junction. A sign indicates SUGARLOAF TRAIL leading west. Follow this good trail as it climbs, contours, drops, and climbs again to the forested 9952' summit of Sugarloaf Peak, 3.5 miles from the start.

Return the same way. Or, with a car shuttle, descend Green Canyon to Forest Road 2N93, 5 miles north of where you left it (Hike 32).

WILDHORSE CREEK

Hike Length: 8 miles round trip; 1400' elevation gain
Difficulty: Moderate
Season: April–October
Topo map: *Moonridge* (7.5')

Features

The fault-carved canyon of Wildhorse Creek descends in an almost straight line from high on the Sugarloaf Ridge to the Santa Ana River. Near the head of the canyon is Wildhorse Spring, feeding the creek that runs full in spring but fades to a lazy trickle by late summer. The creek and the protective shade of the canyon walls nourish a lush forest of Jeffrey pine, white fir, incense-cedar, and several varieties of oak. For the most part, this forest is confined to the canyon bottom, and it stands in marked contrast to the sparse growth of scattered Jeffreys and semi-arid brush that dot the slopes above.

This trip follows a newly built trail up over chaparral-coated ridges and down into upper Wildhorse Creek, superseding the old trail that follows the length of the creek. For an overnight stay there is Wildhorse Creek Trail Camp, nestled amid tall Jeffrey pines and white firs alongside the trickling creek. If you like solitude and nature's peace, this is the trip for you. In summer, when a multitude of hikers tramp through nearby San Gorgonio Wilderness, Wildhorse Canyon is usually left alone. I like it best in April or early May, when the air is crisp, Wildhorse Creek runs full, and Old Greyback sparkles under its snowy mantle.

Description

From Redlands drive east on State Highway 38 to the turnoff of the Wildhorse Trail, on your left just before mile marker 038 SBD 33.40 and 0.2 mile *before* the Heart Bar Campground road. Turn left (north) and drive about 20 yards up a dirt road to a signed parking area (**GPS SB34**).

Follow the well-built trail, which for the first mile is an old jeep track, up through an open forest of Jeffrey and pinyon pine and juniper. From the end of the jeep track, your trail winds steadily upward, over and around several ridges, leaving the forest behind. As you climb higher, snow-streaked Greyback Ridge begins to emerge from behind the forested slope of Grinnell Mountain, and views open up down the broad canyon of the upper Santa Ana River. After 3 miles you finally round the last ridge and then descend into the forested canyon of Wildhorse Creek. Another short mile brings you to Wildhorse Creek Trail Camp, located on a bench above the stream, shaded by tall Jeffrey pines (**GPS WPT SB34A**). The creek usually runs all year, although fading to a trickle by late summer.

From the trail camp, you may retrace your steps. Or you can cross the creek and descend the unmaintained Wildhorse Creek Trail 2.25 miles to State Highway 38 at a bridge at mile marker 038 SBD 31.77 (**GPS WPT SB34B**). This beautiful old trail stays within a few yards of the creek almost all the way down. It is clear for the first mile, then becomes fainter and occasionally brushy before eventually vanishing at the bottom. Arrange a car or bicycle shuttle or plan on a tedious 1.6 miles trudge up the narrow highway shoulder back to the Wildhorse Trailhead.

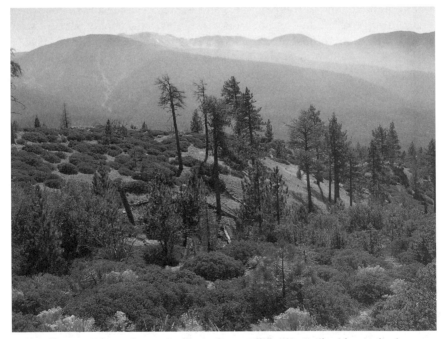

Grinnell Mountain and San Gorgonio from Wildhorse Trail with smoke from forest fire

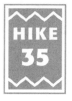

SANTA ANA RIVER HEADWATERS

Hike Length: 9 miles round trip; 800' elevation gain
Difficulty: Moderate
Season: April–October
Topo map: *Moonridge* (7.5'),
San Gorgonio Wilderness (Tom Harrison)

Features

For most of its length from the mountains to the sea, the Santa Ana River is not particularly appealing. Fortunately for hikers and nature lovers, the headwaters of the Santa Ana, close under the forested and gravelly ridges of the San Gorgonio high country, are a delight to behold. The sparkling waters of the new-born river flow through verdant meadows and luxuriant streamside growth, amid a mixed forest of Jeffrey and ponderosa pine, white fir, and black oak.

Description

From Redlands drive east on State Highway 38 to a paved trailhead parking area on your left (**GPS SB35**) just past mileage marker 038 SBD 30.74, 100 feet before the South Fork Campground turnoff to the right.

Your signed trail, 2E03, drops immediately to the river, passes under the highway bridge, and reaches a second trailhead just below the entrance to South Fork Campground. You switchback up the slope and turn east. In 0.5 mile you reach a junction with the Lost Creek Trail, which branches right and climbs around the west slope of Grinnell Mountain to South Fork Meadows, 5.5 miles. You go left and continue eastward, through the forest, with the Santa Ana River down to your left. Continuing east, you enjoy views of 9952-foot Sugarloaf Mountain on the northern skyline, pass several sidepaths leading down to the river, and look down upon the vast expanse of Big Meadows. You pass an unsigned side trail leading down to Big Meadows and on to Heart Bar Campground, but your trail continues east to Forest Road 1N02.

Return the way you came, or arrange for a car shuttle at Heart Bar Campground or Forest Road 1N02 near its junction with 1N05.

FISH CREEK MEADOW

HIKE 36

Hike Length:	5 miles round trip; 650' elevation gain
Difficulty:	Easy
Season:	June–October
Topo map:	*Moonridge* (7.5'),
	San Gorgonio Wilderness (Tom Harrison)
Permit:	San Gorgonio Wilderness Permit required

Features

Fish Creek rises high on the massive slopes of Grinnell Mountain and Ten Thousand Foot Ridge, and cuts a deep swath before joining the Santa Ana River 2 miles east of Barton Flats. This all-year stream is shaded most of the way by a mixed forest of conifers and the largest grove of aspens in the San Bernardino Mountains. Verdant grasses carpet the creekside, particularly at Lower Fish Creek Meadow, an oval clearing where the canyon elbows from northeast to northwest.

This pleasant streamside trip follows the canyon through its middle reaches, where aspens quake in the cool mountain breeze and monkey flowers add a dash of color in early summer. In early autumn, the aspen leaves turn a brilliant golden yellow, in sharp contrast with the surrounding forest.

Description

From Redlands drive east on State Highway 38 to the entrance road to Heart Bar Campground and Fish Creek (1N02) just past the 038 SBD 33.48 mileage marker. Turn right on 1N02, passing the campground entrance to a junction in 1.3 miles. Go right, up 1N05, a fair dirt road, to the signed ASPEN GROVE TRAIL parking area, 2.7 miles from the highway (**GPS SB36**).

Follow the old dirt road that leads southeast down to Fish Creek, 250 yards. You cross the creek and immediately reach the San Gorgonio Wilderness boundary. There are a few aspens here, but to see more of these lovely trees, take the side trail that goes right (northwest) 0.5 mile to Aspen Grove. The main trail passes the wilderness boundary sign and follows a sloping bench paralleling the creek on its west side. You climb gently through a beautiful forest of white fir, interspaced here and there with tall Jeffrey pines and incense-cedar. You pass the small clearing known as Monkey Flower Flat, then climb over a low ridge before dropping down to the creek. In 1.5 miles your trail crosses Fish Creek to the east bank and, 0.75 mile beyond, reaches the grassy clearing of Lower Fish Creek Meadow and a junction with the Upper Fish Creek Trail (see Hike 37).

Return the same way. An option, requiring a car shuttle, is to go left at the junction to the Upper Fish Creek road-head, 0.3 mile (Hike 37).

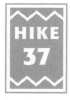

FISH CREEK

Hike Length: 11 miles round trip; 1900' elevation gain
Difficulty: Moderate
Season: June–October
Topo maps: *Moonridge, San Gorgonio Mtn.* (both 7.5'),
San Gorgonio Wilderness (Tom Harrison)
Permit: San Gorgonio Wilderness Permit required

Features

This trip enters the "back door" of the San Gorgonio Wilderness, climbing up Fish Creek and over Fish Creek Divide into the northeastern corner of the wild area. Because driving access is difficult, few hikers use this route. But the forest of pine and fir is rich and green, the waters of Fish Creek are cold and sweet, and the high mountain air is thin and invigorating. For those who wish to linger awhile in upper Fish Creek, there is Fish Creek Trail Camp, with primitive facilities. With a car shuttle, many enjoyable options are available (see below).

Description

From Redlands drive east on State Highway 38 to the entrance road to Heart Bar Campground and Fish Creek (1N02) just past the 038 SBD 33.48 mileage marker. Turn right on 1N02, passing the campground entrance (on your right in 0.2 mile), to a junction in 1.3 miles. Go right, up the fair dirt road 1N05, bearing right at all road forks, to the signed Fish Creek Trail (1W07) parking area, 7.8 miles from the highway (**GPS SB37**).

Walk westward for 0.6 mile on the well-defined trail (avoiding several other less defined paths that lead in other directions), gradually descending, to a new junction with the upper terminus of the Aspen Grove Trail, to your right (see Hike 36). Continue straight ahead as your trail curves southwest into upper Fish Creek. Down to your right, as you near the creek, is a small, inviting trail camp shaded by Jeffrey pine and white fir. The trail then passes through an area of verdant growth, crosses two small side creeks, and climbs along the left (southeast) slope above the main creek, through a rich forest of Jeffrey pine and white fir. After several switchbacks to gain elevation, the pathway contours over into the main draw and reaches Fish Creek Trail Camp, 1.25 miles. The camp consists of several cleared flats amid rocky terrain, shaded by white fir. Water flows year-round in the stream just west of camp.

Beyond the camp, the trail starts climbing the broad slopes of Grinnell Mountain. As it rises above 9000', the view opens to the north and east, over the rugged east-end country of the San Bernardinos and out into the desert.

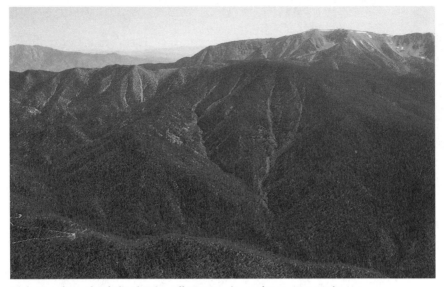

Fish Creek to the left of Grinnell Mountain and San Gorgonio,
with San Jacinto in the distance

Lodgepole pines begin to predominate. After four long switchbacks, you
reach Fish Creek Saddle, on the high divide between Fish Creek and the
South Fork of the Santa Ana, 4.4 miles from the start. A 0.5-mile side trip
north along the crest gets you to Grinnell Mountain for far-ranging views
over the eastern part of the wilderness. (Grinnell Mountain is named for
Joseph Grinnell, 1877–1924, University of California zoologist who made
animal studies in the eastern San Bernardino Mountains during 1905–07.)
From the saddle, the trail contours across the northwest slopes of Lake Peak,
through a forest exclusively lodgepole, toward Mine Shaft Saddle, 0.9 mile
to the Mine Shaft Saddle–North Fork Meadows trail branching left (southeast). Go right (west) 0.25 mile to Mine Shaft Saddle.

Here a number of options present themselves. You can return the way you
came. You can take the Sky High Trail to the summit of San Gorgonio (see
Hike 44). You can descend to Dry Lake and on out to Jenks Lake Road,
requiring a car shuttle (see Hike 42). You can go down the North Fork of the
Whitewater to North Fork Trail Camp (see Hike 45). With several days
available for your outing, you can use this Fish Creek access to visit just
about any part of the San Gorgonio Wilderness you desire.

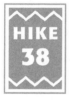

PONDEROSA NATURE TRAIL

Hike Length: 1 mile round trip; 150' elevation gain
Difficulty: Easy
Season: May–October
Topo map: *Big Bear Lake* (7.5')

Features

The Forest Service maintains a number of "nature trails" in San Bernardino National Forest that are designed to inform the visitor of the natural history of the San Bernardinos, pointing out the flora, the fauna, and landscape features. Walking these nature trails, seeing first-hand the various species and features, is the best way to learn nature's story in the mountains.

This short loop trail offers a fitting introduction to the nearby San Gorgonio Wilderness. In a one-mile walk around a hillside and through the forest, you pass examples of most of the flora found in the lower half of the wilderness. Signs are posted every few hundred feet or so, describing what you see. This is a hike you should stroll rather than stride; go slowly, ponder nature's secrets, and you will more fully enjoy your next trip into the San Gorgonio Wilderness.

Description

From Redlands drive east on State Highway 38 to the beginning of the Ponderosa Nature Trail (1E19), marked by a large wooden sign on the left (north) side of the road (0.1 mile before the Jenks Lake turnoff at mile marker 038 SBD 25.51). Park in the adjacent clearing (**GPS SB38**).

The well-graded trail climbs north along the slope, passing and describing various forms of vegetation, turns west and zigzags down into a forested shallow, then ascends southeasterly back to the parking area.

If you return to your car unfulfilled, cross the highway and sample the short (0.6 mile) Whispering Pines Nature Trail (1E33). An interpretive guide to the sights along the trail may be available at the start for a nominal fee.

At the time of this writing, the Ponderosa Trail was closed for repairs but the Whispering Pines Trail was open.

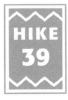

SIBERIA CREEK TRAIL CAMP
FROM SEVEN PINES

HIKE 39

Hike Length: 8 miles round trip; 600' elevation gain
Difficulty: Moderate
Season: All year
Topo map: *Big Bear Lake, Keller Peak* (both 7.5')

Features

This is the back-door approach to Siberia Creek, coming in from the valley of the Santa Ana River. A 1971 fire destroyed much of the forest cover, mainly live oaks and spruces, but trees and other vegetation are slowly growing back. Most of this hike is through open chaparral, exposed to the sun. For this reason, it is best done on a cool winter or spring day when the other approaches—via the Rim of the World Highway (State Highway 18) (Hike 21) and Bluff Lake (Hike 30)—are snowed in. Fortunately, Siberia Creek was spared from the holocaust and is as delightful as ever.

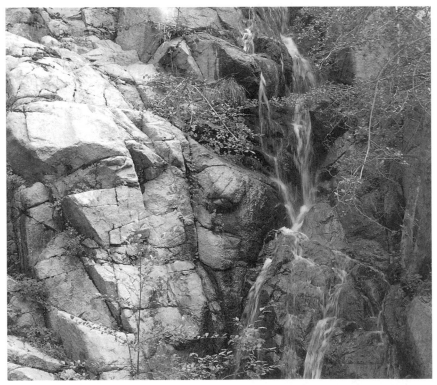

Waterfall along Middle Control Road

The trail was destroyed by rock slides in 2005 and is presently dangerous and not recommended. The Forest Service hopes to send in a trail crew for reconstruction in Spring 2006; contact the Big Bear Discovery Center for up-to-date conditions.

Description

From Redlands drive 19 miles east on State Highway 38 to Angelus Oaks. Just beyond, turn left (north) and descend Middle Control Road (1N06), a good dirt road, crossing the Santa Ana River to reach the Santa Ana River Road (1N09), 3.8 miles. Turn left (west) on the latter and follow it 0.2 mile to a junction with the fair dirt Clark Grade Road (1N54). Turn right and ascend Clark Grade 1.8 miles to a junction with Forest Road 1N64. Turn left (west) and descend. Pass Clarks Ranch Camp and some stream crossings that may be impassible in high water. After 1.7 miles, you will arrive at the Seven Pines Trailhead (1W10), marked by a small sign high above the road on the right. Park in a turnout just beyond (**GPS SB39**). The sign is easy to miss. If you reach a side road to the top of a hill with a good view, you have gone too far.

The first few yards of the trail are badly overgrown and washed out. Follow the trail, overgrown with brush in several places, as it climbs and contours northwest above Bear Creek. In 3 obstacle-filled miles you intersect the new trail coming down from Bluff Lake (see Hike 30). Continue north 1 mile, dropping to Siberia Creek Trail Camp and its welcome shade and water.

Return the same way. Or you have the options mentioned above (see Hikes 21 and 30), both requiring a car shuttle.

SOUTH FORK MEADOWS

HIKE 40

Hike Length: 9 miles round trip; 1600' elevation gain
Difficulty: Moderate
Season: May–October
Topo map: *Moonridge* (7.5'),
San Gorgonio Wilderness (Tom Harrison)
Permit: San Gorgonio Wilderness Permit required

Features

There is only one designated wilderness area in the San Bernardino Mountains. But for multitudes of hikers, it is the grandest in all of Southern California. This is the 35,000-acre San Gorgonio Wilderness, a high mountain wonderland of granite peaks, forests of pine and fir, lush subalpine meadows, sparkling streams and placid lakes, and abundant wildlife. This region is set aside to be preserved forever in its pristine state. Here, under an evergreen canopy, alongside a singing stream or limpid pool, or high on a wind-washed ridge, you can find solitude and freedom, away from the civilization so near yet seemingly a world away. The nourishment afforded by true wilderness should redeem and revitalize you. South Fork (also called Slushy) Meadows, on the north side of the wilderness, is fed by a multitude of springs. It was overused in the past, but is regaining its former glory. Casual hikers going only 2.25 miles to the wilderness boundary do not need a permit. If you're proceeding beyond, to South Fork Meadows, you will need a wilderness permit, available at the Mill Creek Ranger Station, on State Highway 38 a mile below the mouth of Mill Creek Canyon.

Description

From Redlands drive east on State Highway 38 to the Jenks Lake Road turnoff, 50 yards before mile marker 038 SBD 25.51. Turn right (southeast) and follow Jenks Lake Road 2.5 miles to the new, well-marked South Fork Trailhead (**GPS SB40**). There is a large paved parking area with restrooms on your left.

Follow the well-built, easy-graded trail (1E04) as it winds up through stands of Jeffrey pine and white fir, passing the broad expanse of Horse Meadow, to the wilderness boundary at Poopout Hill, 2.4 miles and 1000 feet of elevation gain. You contour eastward along the richly forested hillside, and after another mile begin to hear the rushing waters of the Santa Ana's South Fork down to your left. The trail climbs 200 feet in the last 0.25 mile and reaches South Fork Meadows, a sloping glen shaded by pine and fir, with lush ferns and grasses sprouting along the several converging streams and in the marshy cienegas.

Due to overuse, overnight camping in the South Fork Meadows area has been suspended indefinitely. Picnicking and day use are still allowed. Please take out everything you bring in.

Trails lead southwest to Dollar Lake (see Hike 41) and southeast to Dry Lake (Hike 42) and on to the summit of San Gorgonio Mountain (Hikes 43 and 44). But this particular trail walk ends here at South Fork Meadows; so after enjoying your stay, return the way you came.

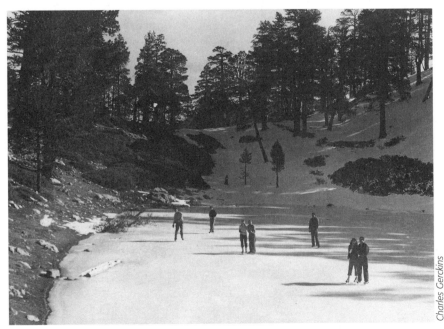

DOLLAR LAKE

HIKE 41

Hike Length:	13 miles round trip; 2400' elevation gain
Difficulty:	Moderate (2 days), Strenuous (1 day)
Season:	June–October
Topo map:	*Moonridge, San Gorgonio Mtn.* (both 7.5'), *San Gorgonio Wilderness* (Tom Harrison)
Permit:	San Gorgonio Wilderness Permit required

Features

High under the north face of the Greyback–San Bernardino Peak ridge, tucked snuggly against rockbound slopes, is the tiny jewel called Dollar Lake. The little circular lake was so named because, when viewed from above on a sunny day, it shines like a silver dollar. Surrounding the lake is a healthy forest of lodgepole pine and white fir. In the trees, along the west shore, is Dollar Lake Trail Camp, one of the most popular and heavily used in the San Gorgonio Wilderness.

This trip follows the well-traveled pathway from Jenks Lake Road to Dollar Lake, where you may picnic but not camp. Overnight camping is allowed at Dollar Lake Forks, just northwest of the lake.

Ice skating on Dollar Lake in 1949

Charles Gerckins

Description

From Redlands drive east on State Highway 38 to the Jenks Lake Road turnoff, 50 yards before mile marker 038 SBD 25.51. Turn right (southeast) and follow Jenks Lake Road 2.5 miles to the new, well-marked South Fork Trailhead (**GPS SB40**). There is a large paved parking area with restrooms on your left.

Follow the excellent trail from Jenks Lake Road to South Forks Meadows, 4.6 miles (see Hike 40). The trail then skirts the west edge of the meadow for 100 yards and begins switchbacking up the ridge. You start out in a forest of ponderosa pine and white fir, but as you climb above 8800 feet, lodgepoles begin to predominate. The trail then rounds the ridge and climbs along the west slope of the big draw leading to Dollar Lake Saddle, passing a grassy cienega, and entering an area of waist-high manzanita. About 1.75 miles above South Fork Meadows, you reach a junction; go left on 1E03, dropping into the bowl above Dollar Lake. In 200 yards you reach another junction; again go left, and follow the trail down to the lake, 0.25 mile. The new trail camp is located 0.25 mile above (northwest of) the lake, adjacent to the junction of the Dollar Lake Saddle and Dollar Lake trails.

Return the way you came. An alternative is to take the old, unmaintained trail that drops directly down the draw to South Fork Meadows: a shortcut, but overgrown and hard to locate in spots. Another option is to climb San Gorgonio Mountain from here, making it an easy two-day trip rather than a strenuous one-day scramble (see Hike 43).

DRY LAKE

HIKE 42

Hike Length: 13 miles round trip; 2300' elevation gain
Difficulty: Moderate (2 days), Strenuous (1 day)
Season: June–October
Topo map: *Moonridge, San Gorgonio Mtn.* (both 7.5'),
San Gorgonio Wilderness (Tom Harrison)
Permit: San Gorgonio Wilderness Permit required

Features

Dry Lake sits in a great amphitheater, surrounded on three sides by the lofty horseshoe crest of Grinnell, Lake, San Gorgonio, and Jepson peaks. The lake is shallow, and in seasons of light precipitation, it dries up by midsummer—hence the name. But in early summer, after abundant rainfall, Dry Lake is full to the brim, and it beautifully mirrors the high granite ridges that soar above it. The forest cover on the surrounding slopes is almost exclusively lodgepole pine, with low clumps of chinquapin here and there. Dominated by the steep, grey-granite face of San Gorgonio, which is often snow-lined into midsummer, this delectable mountain basin approaches true alpine conditions and bears a striking resemblance to the High Sierra.

An excellent, easy-graded trail climbs from South Fork Meadows into Dry Lake basin, where two trail camps have been placed by the Forest Service—one just above the north shore of the lake, the other 0.25 mile beyond at Lodgepole Spring. For those who desire a small taste of the Sierra Nevada close to home, this is an ideal trip. Bring warm clothing and a good sleeping bag if you are going to stay overnight: nights can be nippy at 9000 feet.

Description

From Redlands drive east on State Highway 38 to the Jenks Lake Road turnoff, 50 yards before mile marker 038 SBD 25.51. Turn right (southeast) and follow Jenks Lake Road 2.5 miles to the new, well-marked South Fork Trailhead (**GPS SB40**). There is a large paved parking area with restrooms on your left.

Follow the trail from Jenks Lake Road to South Fork Meadows, 4.6 miles (see Hike 40). Leave the main trail here, which continues up to Dollar Lake and Dollar Lake Saddle (see Hike 41), and cross to the southeast side of the meadows on any one of several beaten paths (a sign points to Dry Lake). Pick up the Dry Lake Trail (1E05) just past South Fork Meadows Trail Camp and follow it southeast into a draw. After about 100 yards, the trail turns left (northeast) and crosses the small stream coming down from Dry Lake basin. It then switchbacks up the mountainside through open stands of ponderosa and Jeffrey pine and white fir. After gaining 400', the switchbacks end and your trail contours along the slope until it rejoins the floor of the draw. A short distance up the draw it reaches Dry Lake—1.75 miles from South Fork Meadows. Here is a trail junction: right to Mine Shaft Saddle and San Gorgonio Mountain (see Hike 44), left to the two trail camps. You go left. In 0.1 mile the trail reaches Dry Lake Trail Camp, located in a grassy area surrounded by lodgepoles just above the northeast shore of the lake. A quarter mile farther, just inside the draw southeast of Dry Lake, is Lodgepole Spring Trail Camp, with water trickling from the small spring.

Return the way you came. Options include going on up San Gorgonio Mountain (Hike 44) and returning via Dollar Lake Saddle (Hike 43), making a grand loop trip around the eastern part of the Wilderness, or taking the new trail across the ridge to Fish Creek (Hike 37). Any way you do it, you will enjoy this alpine section of the highest wilderness in Southern California.

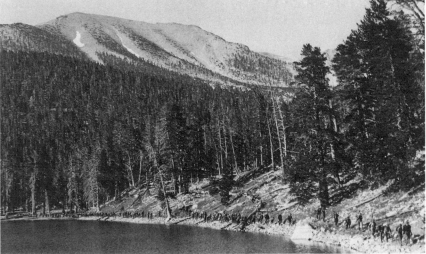

Hikers wind around Dry Lake—San Gorgonio Mountain is in the background (circa 1923)

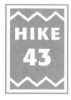

SAN GORGONIO MOUNTAIN
VIA DOLLAR LAKE SADDLE

HIKE 43

Hike Length: 22 miles round trip; 4700' elevation gain
Difficulty: Strenuous (1 day), Moderate (2 days)
Season: June–October
Topo maps: *Moonridge, San Gorgonio Mtn.* (both 7.5'),
San Gorgonio Wilderness (Tom Harrison)
Permit: San Gorgonio Wilderness Permit required

Features

San Gorgonio Mountain crowns all of Southern California. No other peak
south of the Sierra Nevada rises high enough to challenge its 11,502' elevation. Gleaming white in winter snows and somber grey during summer
months, its massive granite bulk can be seen for a hundred miles in many
directions.

The great hogback mountain is the culminating hump of the 10,000'-
plus, 7-mile long, sky-piercing ridge that dominates the San Gorgonio
Wilderness. Gravelly, boulder-strewn slopes and broad, shallow draws slant
downward from the summit crest, dropping far into shadowy canyons. Snow
patches linger well into the summer months. The air is crisp with the chill
of elevation. The sky is deep blue, free of the urban-generated murkiness
that clogs lower elevations.

Although a familiar sight to millions living below, only the hiker or horseback rider can really know the charm of this alpine island in the sky. What
look like barren, lifeless slopes from the distance are spotted with hardy,
weather-resistant life-forms. Wind-buffeted dwarf lodgepole pines and limber pines hug the ground between boulders. Small clumps of high altitude
chinquapin sprout in protected hollows. Diminutive alpine wildflowers
bloom colorfully in midsummer—most common are pink-flowered
locoweed, alpine buttercup and silver mat. Golden-mantle ground squirrels
and grayish lodgepole chipmunks dart among the elfin trees. Red-tailed
hawks and Clark's nutcrackers are occasionally seen flying above. Just east
of the summit, on desert-facing slopes, dwell a handful of Nelson bighorn
sheep.

The mountain received its name from Rancho San Gorgonio, the easternmost cattle ranch of Mission San Gabriel, established sometime before 1824
(located in today's San Gorgonio Pass). The rancho, in turn, was named for
Saint Gorgonius, an obscure Christian martyr of the third century A.D. whose
feast day is September 9th. But for many years, the mountain was known by
other titles. The Cahuilla people called it "Kwiria-Kaich," meaning "bald" or
"smooth." Lieutenant Robert S. Williamson's Pacific Railroad Survey party of

1853 were the first to describe the mountain and called the whole ridge "Mount San Bernardino." In 1878 the U.S. Army's Wheeler Survey saw in the great grey hogback a resemblance to a grizzly bear at rest and labeled it "Grizzly Peak" on their map. From the 1870s on, many San Bernardino Valley residents knew the mountain as "Greyback," a name that persists today. Not until E.T. Perkins, topographer for the United States Geological Survey, surveyed the mountain in 1899 and placed the name "San Gorgonio Mountain" on the government topographical sheet did the latter become commonly accepted as the correct title for the peak.

The earliest known ascent of San Gorgonio Mountain was made by W.O. Goodyear of the California Mining Bureau and Mark Thomas of San Bernardino on June 2, 1872. Their route was up the south slope of the mountain from Mill Creek Canyon. Goodyear toted a mercury barometer to the summit and calculated its elevation at 11,600'—not a bad estimate considering his primitive instrument.

Since then, thousands have made the ascent in all kinds of weather conditions. Charles Francis Saunders, in his classic *Southern Sierras of California,* described a terrifying climb amid lightning, thunder and dashing rain in 1904, in which one person was killed and another dazed by a lightning bolt. Because of the elevation and unstable winds, this type of weather occasionally occurs in the summertime. But most often the weather is clear and cool during the summer months, a welcome relief from the sweltering valley far below.

In 1875, Theodore Van Dyke proclaimed "He who has not ascended Grayback is like a savage who listens to the tuning up of an orchestra and goes off pleased—thinking he has heard the concert." This is a trip every Southern California hiker should make at least once. The trail is in excellent condition, the high-altitude atmosphere is invigorating, the alpine life forms offer a striking change from the usual southern California pattern, and the view from the top encompasses a 360-degree panorama from the Mexican border to the southern Sierra Nevada, from the Pacific to the farthest reaches of the Mojave Desert.

You have a number of options. You can do it up and back in one strenuous day. You can make it an overnight backpack by staying at one of several inviting trail camps. Or, with a car shuttle, you can go up this way and descend by another route. All of these options are outlined below.

Description

From Redlands drive east on State Highway 38 to the Jenks Lake Road turnoff, 50 yards before mile marker 038 SBD 25.51. Turn right (southeast) and follow Jenks Lake Road 2.5 miles to the new, well-marked South Fork Trailhead (**GPS SB40**). There is a large paved parking area with restrooms on your left.

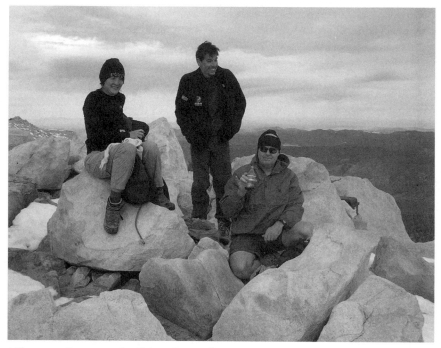

Hikers on the summit of San Gorgonio

Follow the trail from Jenks Lake Road to South Fork Meadows, 4.6 miles (see Hike 40). The trail then climbs above the west edge of the meadow and begins switchbacking up the ridge. You start out in a forest of ponderosa pine and white fir, but as you rise above 8800' lodgepoles begin to predominate. The trail then rounds the ridge and climbs along the west slope of the big draw leading to Dollar Lake Saddle, passing a grassy cienega and an area of waist-high manzanita. Just beyond, you pass the junction of the trail going down to Dollar Lake.

Continue up the trail to Dollar Lake Saddle (**GPS SB43B**, 10,000'), 2.5 miles from South Fork Meadows. Two small trail camps are just west of the saddle: Red Rock Flat (no water) and, 0.5 mile farther west, just south of the main divide trail, High Meadow Springs (always water), both shaded by lodgepole pines. If you are doing the trip in two days, stay overnight at one of these trail camps. Trails lead northwest along San Bernardino Peak Divide (see Hike 49), southwest down Falls Creek to Mill Creek Canyon (see Hike 52), and southeast to San Gorgonio Mountain. You turn left and take the latter trail. The pathway leads through a silent, stony forest of lodgepoles around the west and south slopes of Charlton Peak. In 0.5 mile you reach the steep sidetrail up to Charlton's summit (Charlton Peak is named for Rushton Charlton, supervisor of Angeles National Forest from 1907 to 1925, when the San Bernardinos were part of the Angeles). At 0.7 mile beyond the junction, the trail reaches the saddle between Charlton and Jepson peaks, where you can look down into Dry Lake basin. Here is Dry Lake View Trail Camp, a small overnight stop amid stunted lodgepoles and granite boulders, waterless. The trail now climbs the treeless west slope of Jepson Peak (named for Willis Linn Jepson, 1867–1946, University of California botanist who made a botanical survey of the San Bernardino Mountains in the early 1900s and wrote *Trees of California* and *A Manual of Flowering Plants*), contours high on the south side through dwarfed and windbent lodgepoles, and reaches a junction with the Vivian Creek Trail in two miles (see Hike 54). Continue upward and eastward. About 0.25 mile farther is a second junction, this one with the Sky High Trail leading down around the east slope of the mountain to Mine Shaft Saddle (see Hike 44). The trail now crosses nearly bare slopes, passes the top of Big Draw, crosses a slight rise, and climbs to the boulder-stacked summit of San Gorgonio Mountain, 11 miles from the start (**GPS SB43A**). Adjacent is Summit Trail Camp—no trees, no water, exposed to the elements, but a favorite of hardy backpackers who relish the mountaintop sunrise and don't mind below-freezing temperatures (a Southern California counterpart of sleeping on Mt. Whitney's summit).

After taking in the all-encompassing view, return the way you came. Or you have several options. You can descend by the Sky High Trail to Mine Shaft Saddle and Dry Lake, and back to Jenks Lake Road, a 21.5-mile round trip (see Hike 44). With car shuttles, you can descend the Vivian Creek Trail or the Falls Creek Trail into Mill Creek Canyon (see Hikes 52, 54). Or—very strenuous—you can follow the ridge line trail westward over San Bernardino Peak and down to Angelus Oaks (see Hike 49). Any way you decide to do the trip, you will thoroughly appreciate this sky-reaching part of Southern California.

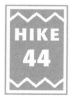

SAN GORGONIO MOUNTAIN
VIA MINE SHAFT SADDLE

Hike Length: 23 miles round trip; 4700' elevation gain
Difficulty: Strenuous (1 day), Moderate (2 days)
Season: June–October
Topo maps: *Moonridge, San Gorgonio Mtn.* (both 7.5'),
San Gorgonio Wilderness (Tom Harrison)
Permit: San Gorgonio Wilderness Permit required

Features

The Sky High Trail zigzags up the northeast and east slopes of San Gorgonio Mountain from Mine Shaft Saddle. When combined with the standard trail route from Dollar Lake Saddle, it makes for an ideal loop trip. You can go up one way and down the other, covering a good part of the unspoiled alpine country in the eastern half of the San Gorgonio Wilderness. The main attraction of the Sky High Trail is the superb view down over the Coachella Valley; on a clear day you can see to the Salton Sea and beyond. Be in top shape for this one, particularly if you plan to hike it in one day. It is more enjoyable as an overnight backpack, camping at Dry Lake or at one of the timberline trail camps.

Description

From Redlands drive east on State Highway 38 to the Jenks Lake Road turnoff, 50 yards before mile marker 038 SBD 25.51. Turn right (southeast) and follow Jenks Lake Road 2.5 miles to the new, well-marked South Fork Trailhead (**GPS SB40**). There is a large paved parking area with restrooms on your left.

Follow the trail from Jenks Lake Road to South Fork Meadows, 4.6 miles (see Hike 40); then the trail to Dry Lake, 1.8 more miles (see Hike 42). If you plan to make this a two-day trip, you may want to camp overnight at Dry Lake, the last available water. Where the trail from South Fork Meadows reaches Dry Lake's outlet is a junction. Go right (south) along the west shore of the little lake, then right again in a quarter mile where path veers off along the south shore to Lodgepole camp. The trail enters a draw, and climbs up the ridge south of the lake, through a forest of almost exclusively lodgepole pine with clumps of chinquapin for ground cover. In 2 miles it reaches Mine Shaft Saddle, on the divide between Dry Lake basin and the desert-draining North Fork of the Whitewater River. Just beyond is a trail junction: left goes down to North Fork Meadows (see Hike 45), and Fish Creek Meadows (Hike 37); right is the Sky High Trail to San Gorgonio Mountain. Go right (southeast); a sign indicates SAN GORGONIO 3.5 MILES. The trail climbs eastward through granite boulder fields and a lodgepole forest, then makes eight switchbacks up the northeast slope of the mountain. You pass the wreckage of a DC-3 that splattered against the mountainside in 1953. Finally, after gaining a thousand feet, the trail rounds the east ridge of San Gorgonio and climbs westward up the south slope. Good views are obtained down into the rugged Whitewater country and beyond to the desert. About 3.25 miles from Mine Shaft Saddle, the trail intersects the main pathway from Dollar Lake Saddle. Turn right (east) and climb 0.25 mile to the summit (**GPS SB43A**).

If you are doing the loop trip, descend via the Dollar Lake Saddle–South Fork Meadows route (see Hike 43). Or return the way you came. Other options include descending into Mill Creek Canyon via either the Vivian Creek (see Hike 54) or the Falls Creek Trail (see Hike 52). Or, very long, follow the crest trail west to San Bernardino Peak and down to Angelus Oaks (see Hike 49).

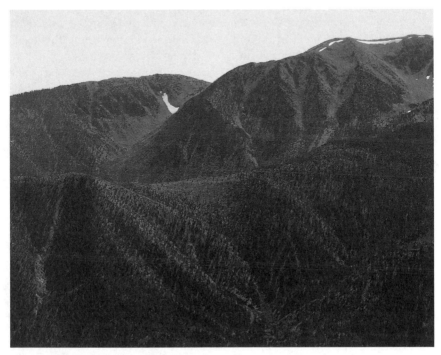

San Gorgonio from the Northeast

NORTH FORK MEADOWS

HIKE 45

Hike Length: 21 miles round trip; 4600' elevation gain
Difficulty: Strenuous (1 day), Moderate (2 days)
Season: June–October
Topo maps: *Moonridge, San Gorgonio Mtn.* (both 7.5'), *San Gorgonio Wilderness* (Tom Harrison)
Permit: San Gorgonio Wilderness Permit required

Features

The eastern end of the San Gorgonio Wilderness drops steeply toward the desert. Draining the 10,000' and 11,000' peaks of this eastern high country are the three forks of the Whitewater River, tumbling streams that through the ages have carved deep, V-shaped gorges from the high mountains down into arid Coachella Valley, where the spent waters sink into the desert sands and the river becomes a broad, gravelly wash. This lower part of the river is the Whitewater known to most people, drab and unimpressive. But the high Whitewater reveals a different character; it is a rugged, isolated wilderness, even today seldom trod by man. Here dwell Nelson bighorn sheep, the largest herds of these noble animals in the San Bernardino Mountains.

Very few trails enter the Whitewater country. One that samples a small bit of it is the overgrown pathway from Mine Shaft Saddle down into the headwaters of the North Fork to North Fork Meadows. Here, alongside the verdant meadow, with Jeffrey pines as a backdrop, the Forest Service has constructed Big Tree Trail Camp. This small campsite, easternmost in the San Gorgonio Wilderness, is well off the beaten track of most hikers. If you relish solitude and quiet beauty on your wilderness outings, this place should be one of your favorites.

Experienced mountaineers have descended the Whitewater all the way to the desert roadend. It is a difficult, trailless venture. Don't do it unless you have done ample cross-country mountaineering, and then never attempt it alone.

Description

From Redlands drive east on State Highway 38 to the Jenks Lake Road turnoff, 50 yards before mile marker 038 SBD 25.51. Turn right (southeast) and follow Jenks Lake Road 2.5 miles to the new, well-marked South Fork Trailhead (**GPS SB40**). There is a large paved parking area with restrooms on your left.

Follow the trail from Jenks Lake Road to South Fork Meadows (see Hike 40), then the trail to Dry Lake, 1.75 more miles (see Hike 42). At the outlet of Dry Lake is a junction; go right (south) and follow the trail up to Mine

Shaft Saddle, 2 miles (see Hike 44). Here is another junction; right up San Gorgonio Mountain (Hike 44), left down into the North Fork of the Whitewater River. Go left (east). The trail gradually descends through a lodgepole forest. In 0.25 mile you pass a trail leading left (northeast) to Fish Creek (see Hike 37); continue straight ahead. Down to your right is Mine Shaft Flats, the scene of an unsuccessful turn-of-the-century mining operation. Just beyond, the trail drops more steeply and leaves the lodgepole forest. You must now fight your way through buckthorn thickets down to the upper edge of North Fork Meadow, 2 miles from Mineshaft Saddle. Here the trail disappears completely and you must thrash through thick brush across the meadow to Big Tree Trail Camp, located under several large pines on the north edge of the meadow. Water runs year-round in the creek, but no wood fires are allowed.

It is easier to approach Big Tree Trail Camp via the unofficial Big Tree track that runs along the northeast side of the creek. This track leaves the official trail below Mineshaft Flat at the head of the ravine that lies on the northeast side of the smaller, upper meadow. It is very hard to find at this point. Work your way down the scree very carefully. You will pick out the track where the terrain levels out. It takes you straight to Big Tree and allows you to circumvent most of the buckthorn that is fast eradicating the regular trail.

The trail ends at Big Tree Trail Camp. Beyond, the Whitewater is wild, and strictly for experienced cross-country backpackers.

Return the way you came. Options include returning over San Gorgonio Mountain (see Hikes 41 and 44) or via the Fish Creek Trail (see Hike 37). The latter requires a car shuttle.

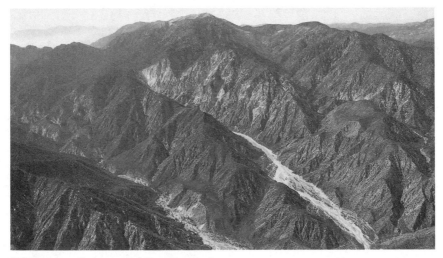

Whitewater Canyon and San Gorgonio

JOHNS MEADOW

HIKE 46

Hike Length: 5.5 miles round trip; 600' elevation gain
Difficulty: Easy
Season: May–November
Topo map: *Big Bear Lake* (7.5'),
San Gorgonio Wilderness (Tom Harrison)
Permit: San Gorgonio Wilderness Permit required

Features

Johns Meadow is a popular family destination for a picnic lunch or easy backpack. It offers a taste of the San Gorgonio Wilderness without the steep climbs required to reach the high mountains. The hike visits lush forest with several small creeks. Quiet hikers will come across squirrels, lizards, and birds. In midsummer, it features wonderful wildflowers and berries, especially where it crosses the creeks. The berries include blue currants (resembling small blueberries with crunchy seeds and a tart taste), small red currants, spikey red gooseberries (tasty if you can get around the thorns), and

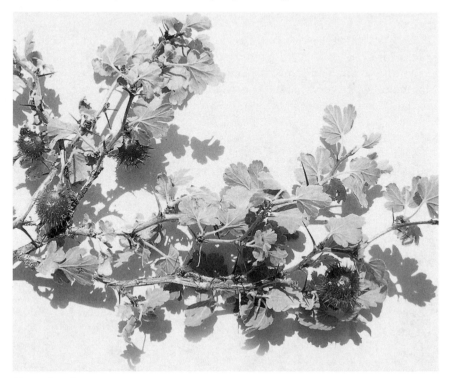

Gooseberries

thimbleberries (red and delicious when ripe, related to raspberries and blackberries). Keep your eyes out for lupine, Indian paintbrush, ferns, and penstemon.

Description

From Redlands drive east on State Highway 38 to the Jenks Lake turn-off, just before mile marker 038 SBD 25.51. Turn right (southeast). After 0.3 mile turn right again onto a fair dirt road where a sign reads FORSEE CREEK TRAIL. Drive 0.5 mile to the large parking area at the trailhead (**GPS SB46**).

The trail starts steeply up the hillside. Pass the Wilderness boundary marker in 0.3 mile. After another 0.1 mile, reach a signed junction. Turn right, toward Johns Meadow. The other path leads to Jackstraw Springs and up to the crest of the mountains (see Hike 48).

The trail now contours westward around the mountainside. It crosses Stetson Creek and another small creek, then climbs gently to a small saddle, 1.8 miles from the junction. Switchback steeply down to Forsee Creek for 0.5 mile. The slope beyond Forsee Creek was scoured by a snow avalanche in 2005, leaving a jumble of twisted tree trunks and debris. 0.1 mile later, arrive at Johns Meadow on a small bench (**GPS SB46A**).

Numerous tent sites are scattered across the bench. The trail becomes ill-defined as it wanders through the sites, but becomes clear again on the southwest side where it crosses another creek. Retrace your steps from Johns Meadow. Or continue up the unmaintained and partially overgrown trail beyond the creek 1.5 miles to Manzanita Springs and on down the San Bernardino Peak Trail to Angelus Oaks (see Hike 48). This requires a car shuttle.

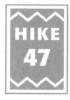

SAN BERNARDINO PEAK DIVIDE
FROM FORSEE CREEK

Hike Length: 18 miles round trip; 3700′ elevation gain
Difficulty: Moderate (2 days), Strenuous (1 day)
Season: June–October
Topo map: *Big Bear Lake, Moonridge* (both 7.5′)
Permit: San Gorgonio Wilderness Permit required

Features

There are numerous opportunities for loop trips in the San Gorgonio Wilderness, laced as the region is with trails. This trip climbs the steep, heavily wooded north slope of San Bernardino Peak Divide via the Forsee Creek Trail, follows the divide trail east to Dollar Lake Saddle, and descends via South Fork Meadows to Jenks Lake Road. En route are several inviting trail camps for overnight stay, and three springs with icy-cold water. You pass through some lush forest country and are rewarded with far-ranging views from high on the 10,000-foot divide. This is one of the best circle trips in the Wilderness. A 3-mile car shuttle is necessary.

Description

From Redlands drive east on State Highway 38 to the Jenks Lake turn-off, just before mile marker 038 SBD 25.51. Turn right (southeast). After 0.3 mile turn right again onto a fair dirt road where a sign reads FORSEE CREEK TRAIL. Drive 0.5 mile to the large parking area at the trailhead (**GPS SB46**).

Leave another vehicle (or bicycle) at the South Fork Trailhead: Continue on Jenks Lake Road 2.2 miles to the new, well-marked South Fork Trailhead (**GPS SB40**). There is a large paved parking area with restrooms on your left.

The Forsee Creek Trail leads uphill through a forest of Jeffrey pine, incense-cedar, black oak, and white fir. In 0.4 mile you reach a trail junction; the fork to the right leads west to Johns Meadow Trail Camp (see Hike 46). Continue straight ahead. In 1 mile you cross little Stetson Creek, trickling water until late summer. A mile farther up, the trail crosses a sloping bench, resplendent with grasses and ferns, spotted with Indian paintbrush and lupine. Beyond, the lodgepole pines begin to appear. Vistas open as the trail rounds the east side of the ridge. As you rise above 8600 feet, lodgepole becomes the predominant forest tree. After 4.5, a sign points right 100 yards to Jackstraw Springs Trail Camp (with wood, water, little flats for sleeping). The trail now climbs the slope east of Forsee Creek and in 2.5 more miles reaches a junction with the lower branch of the San Bernardino Peak Divide Trail, traversing the mountain crest east and west. Just to the right (west) is Trail Fork Springs. Trail Fork Springs Camp (primitive facilities) is on the lodgepole-shaded bench to your left.

Turn left (east); in 0.4 mile you reach a junction with the upper branch of the divide trail (**GPS 47A**), which traverses close under Anderson Peak (named for Lew Anderson, district ranger at Barton Flats during the 1920s). Continue east through a parklike lodgepole forest, around the rocky north slope of Shields Peak (named for Leila Shields, manager of Camp Radford in the 1920s), and down to Shields Flat. There is a waterless campsite here, 80 yards south of the trail. Your trail climbs over a slight rise and drops to a junction with the side trail to High Meadow Spring. The spring and its cozy trail camp are 0.25 mile down the slope to your right (south). Water is always available here.

The trail turns southeast and descends 400 feet to Dollar Lake Saddle, 0.75 mile (**GPS 43B**). Here is a 4-way trail junction and, just to the west, Red Rock Flat Trail Camp (no water). Trails lead southeast to San Gorgonio Mountain (see Hike 43), southwest down Falls Creek to Mill Creek (see Hike 52), and northeast to South Fork Meadows and Jenks Lake Road. Take the latter (see Hikes 38 and 43 for description).

There are numerous ways to vary this loop trip. From Trail Fork Springs, you can turn west along the divide, cross San Bernardino Peak, and descend to Angelus Oaks (see Hike 49). From Dollar Lake Saddle, you can almost double the length of the loop by continuing on to San Gorgonio Mountain (Hike 43), then descending the Sky High Trail to Mine Shaft Saddle, and on down past Dry Lake and South Fork Meadows to Jenks Lake Road (see Hike 44). With a car shuttle, you can descend the Falls Creek trail into Mill Creek Canyon (see Hike 52).

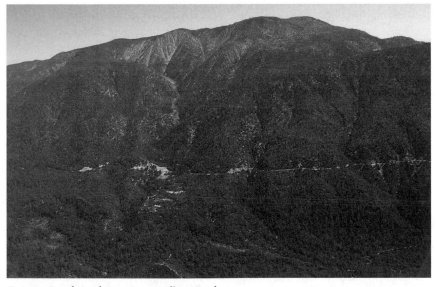

Forsee Creek and San Bernardino Peak

SAN BERNARDINO PEAK

HIKE 48

Hike Length: 16 miles round trip; 4700' elevation gain
Difficulty: Moderate (2 days), Strenuous (1 day)
Season: June–October
Topo map: *Big Bear Lake, Forest Falls* (both 7.5')
Permit: San Gorgonio Wilderness Permit required

Features

The men were exhausted. All day they had struggled up the rugged, trail-less, brush-infested north slope of San Bernardino Peak, all the way from the canyon of the Santa Ana River. The important work they had been assigned to do would have to wait until the next day.

The men were Colonel Henry Washington of the United States Army, under contract with the U.S. Surveyor General's Office; Mr. Gray, deputy surveyor; and 11 workmen. The date was November 7, 1852. Colonel Washington had been assigned the difficult task of establishing an initial point and erecting a monument from which an east-west base-line and a north-south meridian could be surveyed. Then land surveys for all of Southern California would be undertaken, based on Washington's pioneering calculations.

After thoroughly checking the rugged terrain around the peak. Colonel Washington selected a point overlooking the San Bernardino Valley about 0.5 mile west of the summit. Here he and his men erected an elaborate wooden monument 23' 9" in height. Eleven bearings were taken to define the location of the monument, and here the surveyors ran into trouble. They found it impossible to obtain true fixes on distant triangulation marks because of shimmering heat waves from the valley. To overcome this problem, huge fires were lit atop San Bernardino Peak and at the other triangulation points, and the surveys were made at night.

Upon the completion of this initial triangulation, Washington and his party commenced surveying Southern California. All land surveys in this part of the state have subsequently been based on Colonel Washington's base-line.

Today, 150 years later, the wooden base and supporting rock cairn of Colonel Washington's monument remain intact, a few yards above the San Bernardino Peak Trail.

This trail trip visits this historic spot en route from Angelus Oaks to the summit of San Bernardino Peak. You pass through beautiful subalpine country in this western end of the San Gorgonio Wilderness. If the day is clear, views are breath-taking, extending over the foothills and across the vast San Bernardino Valley to the distant San Gabriel Mountains. Two delightful trail camps—Columbine Springs and Limber Pine Springs—offer opportunities for overnight stays. Both have water nearby. It's a long uphill climb, but one you shouldn't miss. Best do it on a cool early-summer or late-fall weekend; long stretches of the trail traverse open manzanita slopes, and are unpleasant walking on a hot day.

Description

From Redlands drive east on State Highway 38 to Angelus Oaks. Follow signs for the San Bernardino Peak Trail (1W07). First turn right from Highway 38 toward the fire station at mile marker 038 SBD 20.00. Then make an immediate left and drive for 0.1 mile, passing the station. Make a right past the station at a sign indicating 1W07 on a fair dirt road. Stay right at two forks and go 0.3 mile to a large dirt parking area with the signed SAN BERNARDINO PEAK TRAILHEAD (**GPS SB48**). The roads to the trailhead have been rerouted recently and may be adjusted again.

The trail starts up through a forest of Jeffrey and sugar pine, white fir, and several species of oak. Soon you are switchbacking up a steep slope. In 2 miles you reach the boundary of the San Gorgonio Wilderness, marked by a wooden sign. A short distance beyond, the switchbacks taper off and you climb more gently through open stands of Jeffrey pine. As you near the top

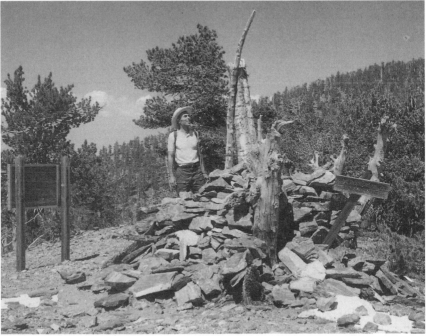

John W. Robinson

Surveyor Colonel Washington's initial point for measuring base-line on San Bernardino Peak in 1852

of a long 8000' ridge, the Jeffreys become less numerous and the trail slices through oceans of manzanita. At 4.3 miles from the start is the Manzanita Springs junction (**GPS SB48B**) just off the trail to the right (south). A side trail leads south down to Manzanita Springs (trickling water in early season but often dry by late summer) and continues 0.25 mile to Columbine Springs Trail Camp (water until mid-summer, sometimes later). The main trail climbs up a slope covered with manzanita, snow brush and chinquapin, and in 1.4 miles reaches Limber Pine Springs Trail Camp. This campsite, located on a bench shaded by lodgepole pines, is the largest trail camp in the western half of the Wilderness and is a favorite of Boy Scout groups. Water is available from Limber Pine Springs, 0.25 mile up the trail. From the springs, the trail turns south and climbs steadily to the top of the high ridge leading west from San Bernardino Peak. In 1.5 miles you reach the west ridge of San Bernardino Peak and climb eastward. Just 100 yards beyond, 50 feet to the right and above the trail is Colonel Washington's initial base-line monument (**GPS SB48C**). The trail climbs eastward along the ridge and in 0.5 mile passes just north of the summit of San Bernardino Peak. A side trail ascends 150 yards to the 10,649' high point (**GPS SB48A**).

After fully enjoying the tremendous view and signing the summit register, return the way you came. An option is to continue eastward along the San Bernardino Peak Divide Trail (see Hike 49), then descending to Jenks Lake Road or Mill Creek Canyon.

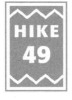

THE GREAT SAN BERNARDINO DIVIDE

Hike Length:	30.5 miles one way; 6200' elevation gain
Difficulty:	Moderate (3 days), Strenuous (2 days), Very Strenuous (1 day)
Season:	June–October
Topo maps:	*Big Bear Lake, Forest Falls, Moonridge, San Gorgonio Mtn.* (all 7.5'), *San Gorgonio Wilderness* (Tom Harrison)
Permit:	San Gorgonio Wilderness Permit required

Features

This long trail trip traverses the entire San Bernardino Peak–San Gorgonio Mountain ridge from west to east, covering a generous part of the San Gorgonio Wilderness. It is for experienced backpackers who relish long stretches of high-altitude walking. This is the rooftop of Southern California, the largest piece of subalpine wilderness south of the Sierra Nevada, delightful summer hiking country, cool and refreshing. But the climb to this sky island is tough, involving over a mile of elevation gain. Be in good condition before you try it.

Description

From Redlands drive east on State Highway 38 to Angelus Oaks. Follow signs for the San Bernardino Peak Trail (1W07). First turn right from Highway 38 toward the fire station at mile marker 038 SBD 20.00. Then make an immediate left and drive for 0.1 mile, passing the station. Make a right past the station at a sign indicating 1W07 on a fair dirt road. Stay right at two forks and go 0.3 mile to a large dirt parking area with the signed SAN BERNARDINO PEAK TRAILHEAD (**GPS SB48**). The roads to the trailhead have been rerouted recently and may be adjusted again. The trip ends at the South Fork Trailhead on Jenks Lake Road, so shuttle another car (or bicycle) there: Continue east on State Highway 38 to the Jenks Lake Road turnoff, 50 yards before mile marker 038 SBD 25.51. Turn right (southeast) and follow Jenks Lake Road 2.5 miles to the new, well-marked South Fork Trailhead (**GPS SB40**). There is a large paved parking area with restrooms on your left.

Follow the San Bernardino Peak trail 4.3 miles to the Manzanita Springs junction, then another 1.4 to Limber Pine Springs Trail Camp. (If you are doing the trip in the recommended 3 days, a first-night stop at Limber Pine Springs Trail Camp is suggested.) Proceed 2.4 miles farther to San Bernardino Peak (see Hike 48).

From San Bernardino Peak, the San Bernardino Peak Divide Trail leads east along or just north of the ridgetop, through an open forest of lodgepole

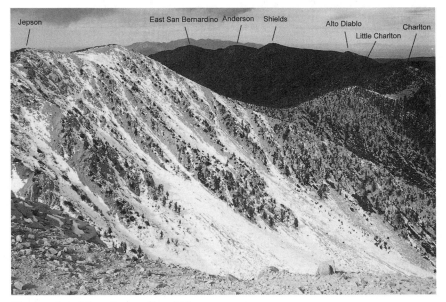

The peaks of San Bernardino Ridge

pine. You drop 200' to a saddle, then climb up the slopes of San Bernardino East Peak, passing just north of the summit (10,691'). A side trail leads 100 feet to the top. About 0.25 mile beyond you pass the unmarked junction of the Momyer Creek Trail coming up from Mill Creek Canyon (see Hike 50, **GPS 50A**). In another 0.5 mile is a trail fork: left to Trail Fork Springs and a junction with the Forsee Creek Trail (see Hike 47, **GPS SB47A**), right for a traverse close under the slopes of Anderson Peak. The two forks rejoin after a mile. Almost pure stands of lodgepole pine cover the ridge from San Bernardino Peak eastward to the upper slopes of San Gorgonio. These hardy veterans of high elevations lack the sylvan greenery and underbrush of lower levels, forming a strange, open, stone-floored forest. Among them a profound silence reigns, occasionally broken by the rat-tat-tat of white-headed woodpeckers and the shrill chatter of chickadees, while toward evening the vesper-like antiphony of hermit thrushes is often heard.

The trail rounds the rocky slope of Shields Peak, drops to Shields Flat, crosses a rise and reaches the High Meadow Springs Trail junction. The springs and trail camp are 0.25 mile to your right (south). The water here is the last before the climb of San Gorgonio, so fill canteens. (If you're doing the 3-day trip, a second night stay here is suggested.) The trail then descends to the 4-way junction at Dollar Lake Saddle, 0.75 mile (**GPS SB43B**). Continue southeastward along the divide trail, rounding the south slopes of Charlton Peak to Dry Lake View Trail Camp (no water) then up around the bare slopes of Jepson Peak and on to the rocky summit of San Gorgonio

(**GPS 43A**), 4 miles, and 18.3 miles from the start (see Hike 43 for detailed description).

You have now traversed the great San Bernardino Peak–San Gorgonio Mountain ridge. After taking in the summit view that encompasses half of Southern California, retrace your steps 0.25 mile to the Sky High Trail junction. Turn left (southeast) and follow the Sky High Trail down to Mine Shaft Saddle, then on down past Dry Lake and South Fork Meadows to trip's end at Jenks Lake Road. This sky-high ramble is the longest in the wilderness, but the spectacular subalpine country you traverse makes the trip well worth the effort.

Alternatively, from Mine Shaft Saddle, descend east on the Fish Creek Trail to the Fish Creek Trail parking area (see Hike 37). This variation shaves off three miles and 1100' of knee-pounding descent, while taking you across the entire San Gorgonio Wilderness from west to east. It requires a longer car shuttle.

The Nine Peaks Challenge is another variation on this trip, climbing all nine summits along the ridge. The San Gorgonio Wilderness Association sells an "I Climbed the Nine Peaks" arm patch. For many Boy Scouts, this three day backpacking trip is a rite of passage. Serious peakbaggers and ultramarathoners attempt it in one exhausting day. The nine peaks are, from west to east:

• San Bernardino Peak	10,649'	(**GPS SB48A**)
• San Bernardino Peak East	10,691'	(**GPS SB49A**)
• Anderson Peak	10,864'	(**GPS SB48B**)
• Shields Peak	10,701'	(**GPS SB49C**)
• Alto Diablo	10,563'	(**GPS SB49D**)
• Charlton Peak	10,806'	(**GPS SB49E**)
• Little Charlton Peak	10,696'	(**GPS SB49F**)
• Jepson Peak	11,205'	(**GPS SB49G**)
• San Gorgonio Mountain	11,502'	(**GPS SB43B**)

SAN BERNARDINO PEAK DIVIDE
FROM MILL CREEK

Hike Length: 14 miles round trip; 5200' elevation gain
Difficulty: Very Strenuous
Season: June–October
Topo maps: *Forest Falls, Big Bear Lake* (both 7.5'),
San Gorgonio Wilderness (Tom Harrison)
Permit: San Gorgonio Wilderness Permit required

Features

From the faultline gorge of Mill Creek Canyon, San Bernardino Peak Divide rises precipitously over a mile above. This is one of the highest and steepest mountain walls in the San Bernardinos. Climbing directly up this towering slope in seemingly endless-switchbacks is the Momyer Creek Trail, gaining 5000' in 7 miles. The trip presents a living demonstration of how the forest changes with altitude: first through brush and oak, then through belts of Jeffrey and ponderosa pine and white fir, then across manzanita slopes, and finally into the realm of lodgepole pine. There is no dependable water en route, unless you make the 2-mile round trip to Alger Creek. This is a very steep trip for the well-conditioned hiker. Do it on a cool day, and get an early start, for much of the trail is open to the sun. The upper portion is not maintained, but is generally possible to follow. Wear long pants to fend off the brush. You will probably have the trail to yourself; few hikers use this tough route to the high country,

Description

From Redlands drive east on State Highway 38 to its junction with Valley of the Falls Road at the huge switchback 20 yards before mile marker 038 SBD 15.00. Turn right and continue east up Mill Creek Canyon to the large parking area for the Momyer Creek and Falls Creek trails, on your left 100 yards before the fire station, 2.9 miles (**GPS SB50**). Mill Creek Canyon is prone to dangerous mudslides and avalanches in times of heavy precipitation and hiking is not recommended on those days.

Follow the trail down into the broad-shouldered wash of Mill Creek. The trail across the creek washes out every winter so some routefinding is necessary. Go left at a hard-to-spot junction and traverse directly across the boulder maze to the north bank. Here the trail turns left (west) and climbs the open slope to a junction with the old beginning of the Momyer Creek Trail coming up from Torrey Pines Road. Turn right and follow the footpath as it switchbacks steeply up the divide between Momyer Creek and Alger Creek, through chaparral and scrub oak. Soon you are climbing through a patchy forest of oak and Jeffrey pine. In 2.5 miles you reach a junction: a trail right goes 1 mile to Alger Creek Trail Camp (see Hike 51); you go left. Long switchbacks continue and the forest becomes richer—mostly Jeffrey and ponderosa pine and white fir. In 4.5 miles the trail steepens and you cross slopes blanketed with manzanita, and some patches of snow brush and chinquapin. You cross over the sharp south ridge of San Bernardino East Peak, pass more manzanita, and finally enter an open lodgepole forest. One final switchback gets you to the top of the divide 0.5 mile east of San Bernardino East Peak, where you meet the San Bernardino Peak Divide Trail (see Hike 49), 7 miles from the start (**GPS SB50A**).

You now have a number of options. You can return the same way. You can follow the divide trail west over San Bernardino Peak and down to Angelus Oaks (see Hike 48). You can take the divide trail east to Dollar Lake Saddle (see Hike 49), then down the Falls Creek Trail (see Hike 52) to Mill Creek Canyon, reaching the latter 0.5 mile east of the Momyer Creek Trail roadhead, making a 19-mile loop trip without a car shuttle. These are the most practical options; others will reveal themselves if you study the map.

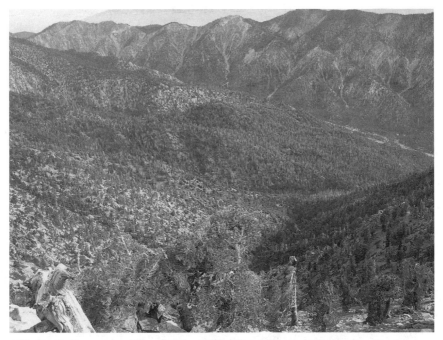

Mill Creek Canyon and the Yucaipa Ridge from the San Bernardino Peak Divide

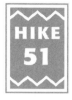

ALGER CREEK TRAIL CAMP

HIKE 51

Hike Length: 6.5 miles round trip; 1400' elevation gain
Difficulty: Moderate
Season: June–October
Topo map: *Forest Falls* (7.5'),
                   San Gorgonio Wilderness (Tom Harrison)
Permit: San Gorgonio Wilderness Permit required

Features

Alger Creek rises high on San Bernardino Peak Divide and flows steeply down the south slope into Mill Creek Canyon. Deeply recessed into the mountainside, shaded by rich stands of pine, fir, cedar, and alder, the little creek seldom suffers the full glare of sunlight. It is a delightful place to relax and keep cool and enjoy nature's sylvan charms on a hot summer day. The Forest Service has built a beautiful trail camp on a bench shaded by tall incense-cedars, just above the churning waters of Alger Creek.

This formerly was a loop trip, until a property owner's complaint cowed the Forest Service into closing the lower portion of the Falls Creek Trail—in spite of the fact that the trail, built by John W. Dobbs in 1898, has been a public thoroughfare for over 100 years. Now you must go and return via the Momyer Creek Trail.

Description

From Redlands drive east on State Highway 38 to its junction with Valley of the Falls Road at the huge switchback 20 yards before mile marker 038 SBD 15.00. Turn right and continue east up Mill Creek Canyon to the large parking area for the Momyer Creek and Falls Creek trails, on your left 100 yards before the fire station, 2.9 miles (**GPS SB50**). Mill Creek Canyon is prone to dangerous mudslides and avalanches in times of heavy precipitation and hiking is not recommended on those days.

Follow the trail down into the broad boulder wash of Mill Creek. The path across the creek is washed away almost every spring, so there's no use trying to follow it. Instead, traverse directly across the boulder maze to the north bank, where you will pick up a recently constructed trail that climbs north onto a low bench. Here your trail turns left (west) and climbs the chaparral-blanketed slope to a junction with the old beginning of the Momyer Creek Trail coming up from Torrey Pines Road. Turn right and follow the well-defined footpath as it switchbacks steeply up the divide between Momyer Creek and Alger Creek, through chaparral and scrub oak. Soon you are climbing through a patchy forest of oak and Jeffrey pine.

In 3 miles you reach the marked junction with the Alger Creek Trail, branching right (northeast). Turn right and follow this lateral trail, following the line of John Dobbs' old flume, before dropping to Alger Creek Trail Camp, 1 mile. The cedar-shaded trail camp is to your right, just above the tumultuous creek.

Your trail continues 100 yards to the creek, fords it, and continues on to Falls Creek (see Hike 52). But you enjoy the delightful wilderness setting of Alger Creek, then return the way you came.

DOLLAR LAKE SADDLE FROM MILL CREEK

HIKE
52

Hike Length:	17 miles round trip; 4500' elevation gain
Difficulty:	Moderate (2 days), Strenuous (1 day)
Season:	June–October
Topo maps:	*Forest Falls, San Gorgonio Mtn.* (both 7.5'), *San Gorgonio Wilderness* (Tom Harrison)
Permit:	San Gorgonio Wilderness Permit required

Features

The Falls Creek Trail, climbing from Mill Creek Canyon to Dollar Lake Saddle atop the main divide, is one of the historic pathways in the San Gorgonio Wilderness. The lower part of it was constructed by John W. Dobbs in 1898, in order to tap the water of Falls Creek and build a flume for a hydroelectric plant in lower Mill Creek. Unfortunately the Forest Service has closed the lower portion of the trail because of an objection by a property owner in Mill Creek Canyon. Now the only legitimate route into Falls Creek from below is via the Momyer Creek Trail and the Alger Creek Lateral Trail, a roundabout way adding six miles to the round trip. Nevertheless, this trip is an inviting one, reaching into the geographical center of the Wilderness and giving access to three beautiful trail camps—Alger Creek, Dobbs Cabin and Saxton. You can stay the night at one of these trail camps and return the same way, or you can use the route as a springboard for any of several Wilderness loop trips, the best of which are mentioned on the next page.

Description

From Redlands drive east on State Highway 38 to its junction with Valley of the Falls Road at the huge switchback 20 yards before mile marker 038 SBD 15.00. Turn right and continue east up Mill Creek Canyon to the large parking area for the Momyer Creek and Falls Creek trails, on your left 100 yards before the fire station, 2.9 miles (**GPS SB50**). Mill Creek Canyon is prone to dangerous mudslides and avalanches in times of heavy precipitation and hiking is not recommended on those days.

Follow the trail down into the broad boulder wash of Mill Creek. The path across the creek is washed away almost every spring, so there's no use trying to follow it. Instead, traverse directly across the boulder maze to the north bank, where you will pick up a recently constructed trail that climbs north onto a low bench. Here your trail turns left (west) and climbs the chaparral-blanketed slope to a junction with the old beginning of the Momyer Creek Trail coming up from Torrey Pines Road. Turn right and follow the well-defined footpath as it switchbacks steeply up the divide between Momyer Creek and Alger Creek, through chaparral and scrub oak. Soon you are climbing through a patchy forest of oak and Jeffrey pine.

In 3 miles you reach the marked junction with the Alger Creek Trail, branching right (northeast). Turn right and follow this lateral trail, following the line of John Dobbs' old flume, before dropping to Alger Creek Trail Camp, 1 mile. The cedar-shaded trail camp is to your right, just above the tumultuous creek.

Cross the creek and continue east on the Alger Creek Lateral Trail as it climbs, then contours around the steep mountainside to a junction with the Falls Creek Trail, 1 mile. Turn left (northeast) onto the latter. In 100 yards you pass the San Gorgonio Wilderness boundary sign, then climb east through a lush forest of Jeffrey pine and white fir to the ridge just west of Falls Creek. Here is another trail junction. To visit Dobbs Cabin Trail Camp, go right and steeply down to Falls Creek 0.25 mile. Just across the creek is the trail camp, set on little flats and shaded by tall cedars, firs, and pines. Dobbs' old cabin site is at the lower edge of the camp; only log foundations remain. To continue up the main trail, go left at the junction. The trail climbs through open forest along the west slope of Falls Creek, fords the west fork, and reaches Saxton Trail Camp, 2 more miles. Water is available from the west fork, 0.2 mile down the trail. Your trail now climbs northeastward, passes the sloping bog of Plummer Meadow (camping no longer permitted), fords the east fork of Falls Creek, and climbs steeply up through a lodgepole forest to Dollar Lake Saddle, 8.5 miles from the start. Two small

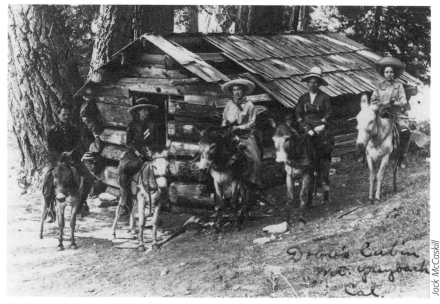

Dobb's Cabin, circa 1910

Jack McCaskill

trail camps are just west of the saddle: Red Rock Flat (no water) and, 0.5 mile farther west, just south of the main divide trail, High Meadow Springs (always water).

You now have a number of options. You can return the way you came. You can turn right (southeast) and ascend San Gorgonio Mountain (see Hike 43), then descend via the Vivian Creek Trail (see Hike 54). You can turn left (northwest) and follow the San Bernardino Peak Divide Trail (see Hike 49), then descend either the Momyer Creek Trail back to Mill Creek Canyon (see Hike 50) or continue on to Angelus Oaks (Hikes 46, 49). Or, turn northeast and descend to South Fork Meadows and Jenks Lake Road (see Hikes 38, 43).

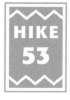

BIG FALLS

Hike Length: I mile round trip; 200' elevation gain
Difficulty: Easy
Season: April–October
Topo maps: *Forest Falls* (7.5'),
San Gorgonio Wilderness (Tom Harrison)

Features

Falls Creek churns and somersaults from high on the shoulders of San Bernardino Peak Divide into a narrow hanging valley, then plunges headlong into the canyon of Mill Creek. The place where it makes this final drop is known as Big Falls. Author-naturalist Charles Francis Saunders described it best: "Looking upward, you see the little creek, a couple of hundred feet above, leap out of a patch of blue sky and drop by a succession of precipitous pitches down a narrow, shadowy gorge, to be shattered at the bottom into a series of musical cascades." Waterfalls are infrequent in the San Bernardinos; it seems a slight upon the beauty of this one that it should have been given no more fanciful name than Big Falls.

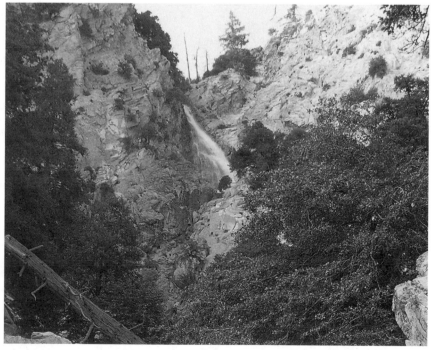

Big Falls

These spectacular falls are but a short walk from the Mill Creek road. Visit them in the springtime, when the melting mountain snowpack is filling Falls Creek, and canyonsides are aroar with the thunder of plunging waters. Bring sandals and a swimsuit.

Description

From Redlands drive east on State Highway 38 to its junction with Valley of Falls Drive at the huge switchback 20 yards before mile marker 038 SBD 15.00. Continue on the latter east up Mill Creek Canyon to the Big Falls parking area on your left, 4.3 miles.

Follow the trail down across the broad boulder wash of Mill Creek, where it disappears among the boulders. The creek crossing may be difficult in times of high water; bring sandals or wading shoes and exercise caution. The trail then climbs into the lower end of Falls Creek to a viewpoint some 200 yards below the falls. Hikers have been injured trying to climb the falls, so do not venture beyond the trail's end.

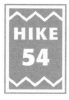

SAN GORGONIO MOUNTAIN VIA VIVIAN CREEK

HIKE 54

Hike Length:	17 miles round trip; 5500' elevation gain
Difficulty:	Moderate (2 days), Very Strenuous (1 day)
Season:	June–October
Topo maps:	*Forest Falls, San Gorgonio Mtn.* (both 7.5'), *San Gorgonio Wilderness* (Tom Harrison)
Permit:	San Gorgonio Wilderness Permit required

Features

The Vivian Creek Trail is the shortest way to climb San Gorgonio Mountain, but also one of the steepest. You start from near the head of Mill Creek Canyon, climb into the verdant hanging valley of Vivian Creek, cross a high ridge into High Creek, and finally ascend gravelly slopes to the barren summit. En route you pass three beautiful trail camps—Vivian Creek, Halfway Camp, and High Creek. Any one of the three makes a pleasant overnight stop if you are doing the mountain in two days.

The Vivian Creek Trail was the first one up the mountain, built shortly after the creation of the San Bernardino Forest Reserve in 1893. For years it was known as "The Government Trail" and was the only one to San Gorgonio's summit. Today it is just one of many but, in the opinion of many hikers, it remains one of the best.

Vivian Creek is a good way to climb San Gorgonio in the winter or spring. An ice axe and snowshoes or crampons are usually necessary. This is a serious route when covered in snow and has recently claimed the life of a solo climber.

Description

From Redlands drive east on State Highway 38 to its junction with Valley of Falls Drive at the huge switchback 20 yards before mile marker 038 SBD 15.00. Turn right and continue east up Mill Creek Canyon to a new parking area on your left, just before reaching closed Big Falls Campground, 4.5 miles. Park at the Vivian Creek Trail sign (**GPS SB54**). Walk on up the dirt road, through the closed campground, to the old trail head parking area, about 0.75 mile.

Follow the trail down across the boulder wash of Mill Creek, then up the mountainside. The first mile is a sharp pull through oak woodlands—unpleasant going if the day is hot—to the secluded hanging recess of Vivian Creek. Here, nestled in a green forest of cedar, fir, and pine, is Vivian Creek Trail Camp, 1.5 miles from the start. The welcome campsites are spread out for several hundred yards near the bubbling creek. Camp at least 200 feet from the water. Beyond, the trail follows the creek, switching from bank to

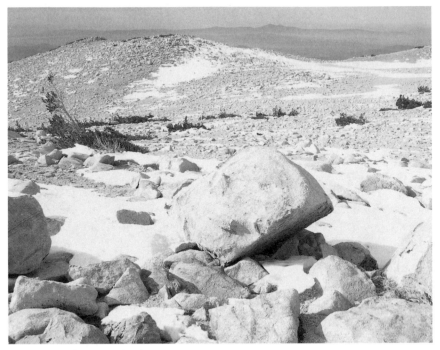

San Gorgonio summit plateau

bank, for another 1.2 miles through miniature meadows spotted with wild-flowers and shaded by tall ponderosa pines and incense-cedars, to Halfway Camp, 3 miles out. This new trail camp has year-round water and many lit-tle flats for sleeping. Beyond, your trail climbs across a ridge to a high-perched, grassy cienega threaded by a small stream of cold, tumbling water. Here is High Creek Trail Camp (**GPS SB54A**), 4.8 miles out, a favorite with backpackers, but the altitude is 9000' and nights are apt to be cold. The pines, cedars, and firs have been left below, and the slopes are covered with almost pure stands of weather-resistant lodgepole pines. The view across the head of Mill Creek Canyon to the saw-toothed wall of Yucaipa Ridge is rem-iniscent of the Sierra Nevada. Above High Creek, the trail winds up through silent lodgepoles to timberline at about 11,000'. Ahead looms the massive crown of San Gorgonio, stark against the deep blue sky. Just below the sum-mit you meet the main trail from Dollar Lake Saddle (**GPS SB54B**); turn right (east) and cross gravelly slopes, passing a few wind-flattened limber pines and diminutive alpine flowers, to the 11,502-foot summit, 8 miles from the start (**GPS SB43A**).

Return the way you came. A popular option is to take the trail west to Dollar Lake Saddle, then descend the Falls Creek Trail back to Mill Creek Canyon (see Hike 52).

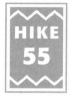

GALENA PEAK

HIKE 55

Hike Length:	9 miles round trip; 3200' elevation gain
Difficulty:	Strenuous
Season:	May–October
Topo maps:	*Forest Falls, San Gorgonio Mtn.* (both 7.5'), *San Gorgonio Wilderness* (Tom Harrison)

Features

Galena Peak at 9324' rises precipitously above the head of Mill Creek Canyon. It is the most rugged-appearing peak in the San Bernardinos, standing in marked contrast to the higher but rounded summits of the nearby San Gorgonio Wilderness. No trails approach its rugged upper ramparts, and you must scramble high over loose boulders and steep rock slopes to stand on its crown.

Part of the Mill Creek headwall has slid away recently, making the trip more tedious than it was a few years ago. You must make a trailless, loose uphill scramble from the head of Mill Creek to the saddle that divides the headwaters of Mill Creek from those of the Whitewater River—known by the curious name of Mill Creek Jumpoff. You need cross-country experience and must wear boots with good tread.

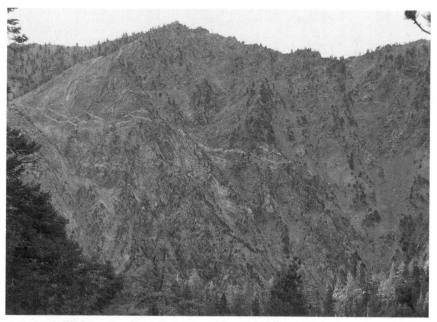

Galena Peak from the north

Description

From Redlands drive east on State Highway 38 to its junction with Valley of Falls Drive at the huge switchback 20 yards before mile marker 038 SBD 15.00. Turn right and continue east up Mill Creek Canyon to a new parking area on your left, just before reaching closed Big Falls Campground, 4.5 miles. Park at the Vivian Creek Trail sign (**GPS SB54**). Walk on up the dirt road, through the closed campground, to the old trail head parking area, about 0.75 mile.

Hike up the poor dirt road that heads east up-canyon. When it ends, continue up the streambed to the headwall at the end of Mill Creek. Climb a small ridge just left of center, then bear right across loose rock slopes to Mill Creek Jumpoff, 4 miles. Turn right (south) and climb up the steep ridge, following a faint climbers' trail part way. Where the trail gets too close to the crumbling headwall, veer left and work your way through manzanita. Approaching the ridgetop, your route veers south-west and divides. The left path climbs to the eastern summit—Galena Peak. The right path climbs to the western summit, slightly higher but unnamed.

Return the same way. Do *not* try to descend directly into Mill Creek Canyon; it is steep, loose, and dangerous.

CRAM AND MORTON PEAKS

HIKE 56

Hike Length:	9 miles one way; 2800′ elevation gain
Difficulty:	Moderate
Season:	November–April
	(fire closure 7/1 to winter rain)
Topo map:	*Yucaipa* (7.5′)

Features

In winter, when the air is crisp and clear and the nearby high country is sparkling white, take this ridgetop walk to Morton Peak Lookout for a rewarding experience. From the 4624-foot summit you get a grandstand vista of the snowy south slope of the San Bernardinos, with 2-mile-high San Bernardino Peak looming massively a few miles to the east. Below, you can trace the course of the great San Andreas Fault straight as a beeline, which forms the southwest and south boundary of the San Bernardinos.

This is a chaparral walk all the way, partly on fire road, but mostly on the ridgetop trail. A car shuttle is required. If you drive the steep 3 miles up the Morton Peak Lookout fire road—sometimes open to the public in winter—the hiking distance is cut to 6 miles. Never, never take this trip on a hot day.

Description

From Redlands drive 5 miles east on State Highway 38 to Greenspot (2 miles past Mentone). Turn left (north) on Garnet Street, which makes two sharp turns and becomes Greenspot Road. Drive 2.5 miles to the unmarked Front Line fire road, on your right (east). Park here outside the locked gate (**GPS SB56**); do not block the gate. If you cross the second Santa Ana river bridge, you have gone too far. You will come out on the Morton Peak Lookout fire road, 2.2 miles east of Mill Creek Ranger Station on State Highway 38, so arranged to be picked up there (**GPS SB56A**).

Walk up the fire road, which turns north, paralleling the Santa Ana River, then east again, to a junction, 0.5 mile. Take the right fork and continue 0.25 mile to the beginning of the Morton Ridge Trail on the left (north), marked by a sign (2w15). Follow the trail as it climbs north to the top of the bare ridge, then east along the ridgetop. In 2.5 miles of steady climbing you round the south side of Cram Peak, just below the 4162-foot summit. The trail then drops 200′ and continues east along the long ridgetop, rounding the north side of an unnamed bump to a spur road, 5 miles from the start. Follow the fire road 1 mile to the summit of Morton Peak (4624′). The fire lookout is permanently closed. After taking in the all-encompassing panorama, descend the Morton Peak Lookout Road 3 miles to State Highway 38.

PART 2

The San Jacinto Mountains

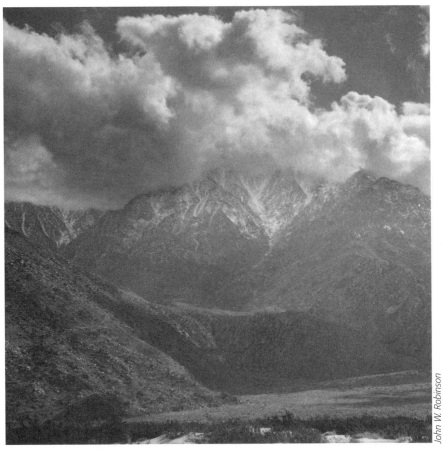

John W. Robinson

Storm over the heights—San Jacinto from the desert

Natural History of the San Jacinto Mountains

Lay of the Land

On clear days, travelers driving through San Gorgonio Pass (also called Banning Pass) toward the desert are treated to an awesome panorama. To their left, dominating the northern skyline, is the abrupt south slope of the San Bernardinos, crowned by the long gray hogback of San Gorgonio Mountain. To their right, and ahead, towers a stupendous rock escarpment, soaring in jagged ridgelines and scoured avalanche troughs almost 10,000 vertical feet in five horizontal miles. This mountain wall is the northeast face of 10,804-foot San Jacinto Peak, as rugged a precipice as exists in the United States. Somber gray in summer and fall, gleaming white in winter, snow-streaked by late spring, San Jacinto's vaulting desert face has fired the imagination and artistry of many a painter and photographer, and awed thousands of desert visitors.

San Jacinto, as is true with most mountains, has its gentle as well as its rugged features. The southwest side of the mountain is made up of rolling hills that rise from the San Jacinto Valley and become progressively higher and steeper until they culminate at the summit. Scenic paved highways traverse this gentle slope, winding through verdant woods, crossing streams that here and there are dammed to provide fishing lakes, giving access to rustic resorts. Idyllwild is the largest and best known of these resort communities, nestled in secluded, mile-high Strawberry Valley.

But it is the summit country of the San Jacintos that is most alluring. Here, well above the highways and byways that penetrate the lower slopes, is a sky island of delectable alpine wilderness, unsurpassed in Southern California. Under white granite summits and boulder-stacked ridges lie little hanging valleys and tapered benches lush with forest and meadow. A multitude of bubbling springs nourishes icy-cold streams that tumble and cascade down the mountain. In season, alpine wildflowers add a beautiful dash of color. The thin atmosphere is cool, clean and refreshing.

Those who confine their mountain exploration to places they can reach by automobile will never see this unspoiled mountain roof-garden. Riders of the spectacular Palm Springs Aerial Tramway can witness a small portion of it. But it is only the hiker or horseback rider who can really know the San Jacinto high country. Summer and fall weekends find hundreds of these outing enthusiasts following the wilderness trails that lace the region, lingering overnight at one of the many secluded trail camps, and climbing to the summit of "San Jack" for a view that is unsurpassed in magnificence. Their numbers are increasing every year.

The top of the San Jacintos are protected from civilization's encroachment by two adjacent wild areas. The heart of the region, including San Jacinto Peak, is included within Mount San Jacinto State Wilderness, under the jurisdiction of the state of California. On both sides of it, north and south, is the San Jacinto Wilderness, part of the San Bernardino National Forest. The recently established Santa Rosa and San Jacinto Mountains National Monument safeguards most of the precipitous desert face of the range.

Geographers disagree over the extent of the San Jacinto Mountains. Some include only the great bulk of San Jacinto Peak and its surrounding ridges and valleys. Others say the San Jacintos take in the whole mountain mass from, roughly speaking, State Route 79, south of Beaumont, southeast some 40 miles to the Palms-to-Pines Highway, beyond which are the Santa Rosas. Most do not include the isolated ridges of Thomas and Cahuilla mountains, southwest of the main mountain mass, although both of these regions are part of the San Jacinto Mountain District of San Bernardino National Forest.

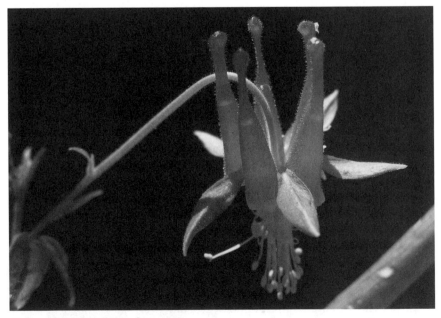

Columbine (*Aquilegia formosa*)

For the purposes of this book, all of the areas mentioned above (except the Santa Rosas) are included in the San Jacinto Mountains.

The geologist looks at the San Jacintos and sees a strong resemblance to the Sierra Nevada. Both are uplifted, westward-tilting blocks, essentially granitic in composition, bounded by major fault zones. He places the San Jacintos in the Peninsular Range province, a line of mountain ranges extending from the Santa Ana Mountains southward to the tip of Baja California. The Peninsular Ranges are generally low mountains, seldom topping 6000′ in elevation. Only the San Jacintos and the Sierra de San Pedro Martir in Baja California rise above 10,000 feet. San Jacinto Peak is the loftiest summit in the entire 800-mile-long province. The San Jacintos are bounded on the west by the San Jacinto Fault, one of the most active in California, the source of many earthquakes in recent years. North and east of the range is a complicated network of relatively short-length faults, offshoots of the great San Andreas Fault. Although not all these desert-side faults have been charted, the stupendous mountain escarpment on this flank bears obvious testimony to their existence.

Plant Life

The botanist studies the San Jacintos and is amazed at the varieties and extremes of plant life. According to Harvey Monroe Hall, whose 1902 botanical survey is still an authoritative source on the flora of the range, "There is probably no place in North America where the alpine and Sonoran floras are in such proximity as they are on San Jacinto Mountain." Between the palm-lined desert canyons at the mountain base and the top of San Jacinto Peak, a horizontal distance of five miles, are stacked all the climatic and vegetation changes one would encounter on a journey from northern Mexico to Canada. Within this short distance are six distinctive life zones, five of which completely encircle the mountain.

At the northeast base, part of the Colorado Desert, is Lower Sonoran vegetation, the most common plants being creosote bush, burro brush, desert willow, and ironwood tree. Above this, in a wide belt extending completely around the mountain, is the Upper Sonoran zone, the principal shrubs being chamise, manzanita, several species of ceanothus and scrub oak, and the main trees being canyon live oak, interior live oak, Palmer oak on the seaward side, and pinyon pine and California juniper on the desert side. The Transition zone embraces the main mountain forest of the San Jacintos, the principal trees being ponderosa pine, Jeffrey pine, Coulter pine, sugar pine, incense-cedar, California black oak, and, higher up, white fir. The Canadian and Hudsonian zones form narrow belts around the higher summits, and are so intermixed that the line between them cannot be definitely drawn. The principal trees—in fact the only trees—of these two zones are lodgepole pine and limber pine, and the main shrub is chinquapin. On the summit of San

Jacinto Peak is a small island of Arctic-Alpine flora, the southernmost limit of this zone in the United States. There are some who question whether the summit is truly Arctic-Alpine, because of the handful of stunted limber pines, Hudsonian zone trees, just below the top. But botanist Hall found several small plants here that definitely are Arctic-Alpine species. Most notable is alpine sorrel, which grows along snow banks just north of the summit.

The climatic extremes are most striking to those living in the Coachella Valley just below the mountain. Winter storms often rage on the cloud-enveloped heights while desert foothills are bathed in sunlight. In early summer, it is not at all uncommon to look up from the sweltering valley floor, with temperatures well over 100 degrees, to see the long fingers of snow glistening in the upper ravines. From the opposite perspective, one can stand high on the northeastern escarpment, shivering from icy blasts of alpine wind, and gaze down on shimmering heat waves rising from the sun-scorched desert.

Wildlife

The wildlife of the San Jacintos is similar to that of the San Bernardinos, and just as timid. Here too, humans have pre-empted most of the range. The most common large mammal is the California mule deer, which summers on the higher slopes and winters at lower elevations. A handful of mountain lions prowl the eastern high country. Bighorn sheep wander on the southern, desert-facing slopes. Bears, once abundant here, are never seen now. On

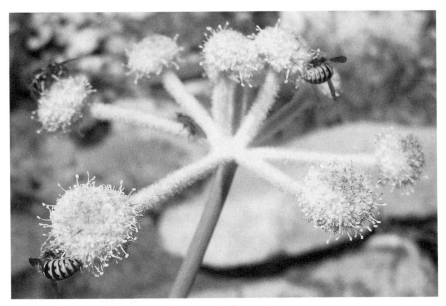

Rangers button (Sphenosciadium capitellatum)

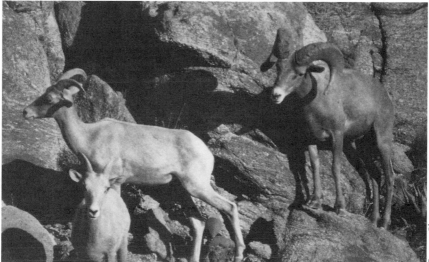

Bonner Blong

Bighorn mountain sheep

rare occasions, the fortunate hiker glimpses a golden eagle soaring over San Jacinto Peak or a high ridge.

Every hiker has a favorite mountain range that never wears out its appeal. To a great many Southern Californians, the San Jacintos are such a range. There are those who return time and time again to sample the rich wilderness offerings of this granite-ribbed island in the sky. And nothing will cure an aggravated case of urbanitis quicker or more thoroughly than a weekend dose of the San Jacintos.

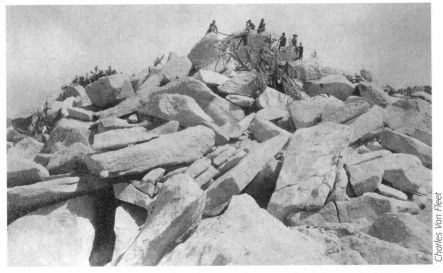

Charles Van Fleet

On San Jacinto's summit — earliest known photograph of the peak, 1885

Human History of the
San Jacinto Mountains

Lure of the Mountains

From this day Ramona never knew an instant's peace or rest till she stood on the rim of the refuge valley, high on San Jacinto. Then, gazing around, looking up at the lofty pinnacles above, which seemed to pierce the sky, ... feeling that infinite unspeakable sense of nearness to heaven, remoteness from earth which comes only on mountain heights, she drew in a long breath of delight, and cried; 'At last! At last, Alessandro! Here we are safe!'

—Helen Hunt Jackson,
Ramona (1884)

This passage, from Mrs. Jackson's wondrous California classic of romance and tragedy, reflects the aurora of reverence and mysticism that has so often been a part of humans' relationship with the San Jacintos. In the novel, the San Jacintos served as a foreboding last refuge for Ramona and Alessandro, Native American lovers, fleeing from the European American's callousness and greed. Mrs. Jackson was not the only famous author to see in these mountains something awesome, enchanting and mysterious. George Wharton James, Charles Francis Saunders, and J. Smeaton Chase all treated the San Jacintos with a degree of reverence unaccorded any other mountains in the Southwest. From their widely read works—and particularly from Helen Hunt Jackson's *Ramona*—the San Jacintos have achieved world-wide fame.

Original Inhabitants
In recent geological history, the Gulf of California reached far into the Coachella Valley to points north of Palm Springs. The Colorado River emptied into the Gulf from the east at about the location of the Salton Sea. Eventually sediment from the Colorado River formed a delta that cut off the

149

north end of the Gulf and formed a lake. This was ancient Lake Cahuilla. Geological evidence of the ancient lake exists today in the form of pebble beach strands and travertine deposits (calcium) on rock outcrops that mark the various shore levels of the lake.

During the existence of Lake Cahuilla, the Colorado River changed course several times, alternately emptying into the lake or the Gulf of California. This and the drier climate caused the lake to alternately dry up and then be refilled. The lake existed from 700 AD to 1400, 1430 to1530, and 1600 to 1700 AD. (Author's note: The Salton Sea was formed in 1905 when the flooding Colorado River overtopped human-made irrigation canals.)

Around one thousand years ago the first humans migrated into the area and inhabited areas along the shores of ancient Lake Cahuilla. These were the Cahuilla Indians and are believed to have migrated from northern Mexico. The Cahuilla survived on an abundance of fish and other sources of nutrition. Archeological evidence of this are the fire rings and stone weirs (fish traps) along the north and northwest shorelines of the ancient lake.

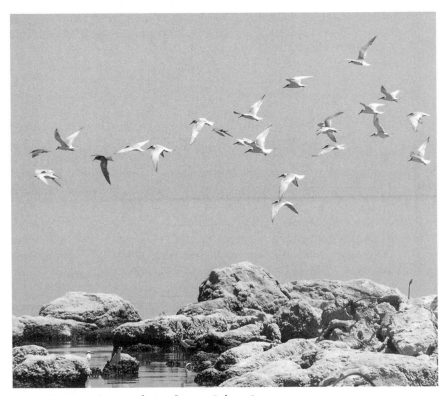

Forster's Terns (*Sterna forsteri*) over Salton Sea

After 1700 the Cahuilla moved into the nearby mountains and canyons where there was a continuing abundance of water and food. Today, the Cahuilla live on the flanks of the San Jacinto and Santa Rosa Mountains. The present day tribes of the Cahuilla consist of the Morongo at the north end of the San Jacintos, the Agua Caliente in the Palm Springs area, and the Santa Rosa in the Santa Rosa Mountains. Other tribes in the area are the Cabazon, Torres Martinez, Ramona, Los Coyotes, and Augustine.

The primary concern of these peoples was the search for food, in which they ranged far and wide. From the desert came such staples as mesquite and screwbean; slightly higher, agave and yucca were collected; and on mountain slopes, acorns and pinyon nuts provided a dependable source of food. Animals hunted by the Cahuillas included the rabbit, wood rat, quail, antelope, mountain sheep, and deer. It was the abundance of deer on the San Jacintos that lured the Western Cahuillas into the high country. Strong hunters climbed the desert face of the mountain to the area where the deer were grazing, killed and dressed them on the spot, and descended with their kill slung over their shoulders.

The Cahuilla Indians were the first to weave a web of mythical lore around the mountains. To the Cahuillas, the San Jacinto Mountains were a sacred place, the home of Dakush, a large, low-flying meteor, legendary founder of the Cahuilla people. They were also the dwelling place of Tahquitz, an evil and powerful demon with an insatiable appetite for beautiful maidens and human flesh. The tales about Tahquitz are many and they vary greatly, but all of them agree that he was a terror to the Native Americans. Hunters and food-gatherers who disappeared in the mountains were said to have been carried off by the evil demon to his lair underneath Tahquitz Peak and eaten. When thunder and lightning rumbled across the mountains, it was said that Tahquitz was angry. At such times, no Native American would dare venture onto the mountain. The Tahquitz legend was known not just to the Cahuillas; it was part of the folklore of almost every Native American people in Southern California.

First Explorers

It was through the Cahuilla Valley and Bautista Canyon, below the southwestern foothills of the San Jacintos, that the early explorers came. First on the scene was the Spanish soldier Pedro Fages, pursuing army deserters from San Diego. Not much is known about the Fages trip, and he left us no descriptions of the San Jacinto country. Two years later, in 1774, came Captain Juan Bautista de Anza, leading a party of 34 from Mexico to Monterey in the most famous overland expedition in California history.

Anza had set out from Tubac, Sonora, to find a route across the desert to California. He and his men almost perished in the burning sands of the Colorado and Borrego deserts, but on their second attempt they managed to find water and locate a gap in the mountain barrier—today's Coyote Canyon. Up this boulder-strewn canyon they struggled until they reached the broad Cahuilla Valley. "Right here there is a pass which I named the Royal Pass of San Carlos. From it are seen most beautiful green and flower-strewn prairies, and snow-covered mountains with pines, oaks, and other trees which grow in cold countries," Anza wrote in his diary. This is the earliest description of the San Jacinto Mountains we have. In the Cahuilla Valley, Anza met 200 peaceful Native Americans—his first encounter with the Cahuillas. Then he descended Bautista Canyon, crossed the San Jacinto Valley, "keeping on our right a high, snow-covered mountain," and continued on to Monterey. Anza passed this way once again in 1776.

Early Settlers, Surveyors, and Prospectors

The Spaniards or their Mexican Californio successors did not settle in the San Jacinto country for many years. Just when they did come to stay is unknown—sometime before 1821 is as close as historians can pin it down. Around this time Mission San Luis Rey established an outlying cattle ranch in the flatlands west of the mountains. This they named Rancho San Jacinto, in honor of Saint Hyacinth of Silesia (1185–1231), a Dominican missionary credited with many conversions in Tibet and China. Thus the name *San Jacinto* was born, first used for the stock rancho, later extended to the San Jacinto Valley, the San Jacinto River, and finally the San Jacinto Mountains.

Except for occasional ventures to search for strayed stock or to hunt grizzlies, the early Spaniards and Californios stayed clear of the mountains. Even with their thick leather chaps, the rancheros found the dense chaparral that coated the lower slopes of the San Jacintos uninviting. There was enough feed for cattle on the plains. The mountains existed mainly as a source of water. There is no evidence that these early Californians ever reached the high country.

With the coming of American and immigrant settlers from the eastern United States—from the 1840s onward—the San Jacintos began to receive more attention. The first believed to have left his mark on the mountains was Tennessee-born Paulino Weaver. Weaver had come to California, perhaps with the Ewing Young trapping party, in the early 1830s. He apparently became a Mexican citizen, for he was granted land in the area of San Gorgonio Pass by Governor Pio Pico in 1845. According to Banning historian Tom Hughes, Weaver was cutting timber from both sides of San Gorgonio Pass—including the northern foothills of the San Jacintos—as early as 1846. He also is said to have hunted bear and deer in the mountains. Weaver later served as a U.S. Army scout during the Civil War, and moved to Arizona, where he died in 1867.

Lieutenant Robert S. Williamson's Pacific Railroad Survey party came through San Gorgonio Pass in 1853. William Blake, geologist of the expedition, crossed to the south side of the pass to investigate the rocks of San Jacinto Peak (which he mistakenly called "San Gorgonio"). His report contains the first scientific description of the mountain.

Lieutenant Williamson's official map, published by the War Department, showed San Jacinto Peak as "San Gorgonio" and San Gorgonio Mountain as "San Bernardino," which for a short time caused confusion among surveyors and new settlers.[1] However, the mistake was rectified two years later (1855) when Lieutenant John G. Parke's Pacific Railroad Survey party passed through the area. Dr. Thomas Antisell, geologist of the Parke expedition, correctly labeled the mountain south of the pass as "San Jacinto," and it has been known singularly by this name ever since.

The 1860s saw pioneer settlers establish isolated homes in the San Jacinto Mountains. Most historians give Charles Thomas credit for being first. Thomas ran away from his New York home at the age of 12, sailed around Cape Horn, landed in San Francisco and drifted south in the 1850s. He took a young Californio bride at Santa Barbara and settled on a ranch near Temecula to raise cattle. The story goes that he was led into the beautiful Garner Valley (then unnamed), high on the south slope of the San Jacintos, by his Cahuilla friends. Thomas fell in love with the mountain-rimmed basin and decided to make it his home. In 1861 he filed on 480 acres in the heart of the valley, brought up his wife and children, and began raising Mexican longhorn cattle there. In 1876 Thomas purchased 4,300 more acres of surrounding mountain land from the Southern Pacific Company. In later years, besides raising cattle, he bred race horses in partnership with Lucky Baldwin. The Thomas Ranch became a well-known Southern California landmark.

To obtain lumber for the ranch buildings and fences, he sent his ranch hands high into the lush forests of the San Jacintos—probably as far as Strawberry Valley—to cut and haul timber. Bears, grizzly and otherwise, abounded in the mountains then. A man named Herkey, cutting timber for Thomas, was attacked and severely mauled while drinking from a creek; he made it back to the ranch, where he died from his wounds. Herkey Creek commemorates him today. Deer were thick in the mountains too. Thomas and his men frequently made hunting trips into the high country. One story tells of deer coming into camp in Round Valley "so tame that six were shot before the herd took fright." Thomas and his family remained on the ranch until 1905, when they sold out to San Bernardino stockman Robert F. Garner.

---

1 Some writers claim that at the same time San Jacinto Peak was called "San Gorgonio," San Gorgonio Mountain was known as "San Jacinto." After extensive research, I was unable to find any evidence of this. As far as can be documented, San Gorgonio Mountain was never known as "San Jacinto."

Others followed Thomas into the San Jacintos—ranchers, herders, hunters, prospectors and lumbermen. As early as 1875, sheepmen and cattlemen herded their hungry livestock into the lush mountain grasslands around Strawberry Valley, some even climbing over the difficult Devils Slide into upper Tahquitz Valley. Hunters soon decimated the large herds of deer. Prospectors searched for mineral wealth in the mountains, but found little to reward their efforts. Henry Hamilton discovered a few valuable tourmaline gemstones on Thomas Mountain in 1872. An Englishman named Harold Kenworthy poured a fortune into a gold-mining operation near the southern end of Garner Valley in the 1880s, but no great amounts of gold were ever uncovered. Emil Chilsen developed the Hemet Belle Mine near Kenworthy around the turn of the century. No one ever made much off the Hemet Belle, and it changed hands so often that it became known as the "Grubstake Mine." Salting mines with gold became a regular procedure: "All you did was load up a shotgun with gold dust, fire it into the rock, and you had a mine for sale," mountain pioneer Lincoln Hamilton recalled.

Timber and Water Seekers

It was the commercial loggers who really opened up the San Jacintos. Rich stands of sugar and ponderosa pine had long been known to exist in the mountains, but the difficulty of hauling out timber over rugged slopes had prevented all but insignificant logging efforts by local settlers. To bring out this timber, wagon roads would need to be hacked up the steep mountainsides. Two such projects were begun in 1875–76: one up the north slopes from San Gorgonio Pass, the other up the west side from the San Jacinto Valley.

It was the Southern Pacific Railroad that got things started on the north side. The Southern Pacific was constructing its main east-west line through San Gorgonio Pass and needed lumber for construction camps and railroad ties. To obtain this timber, Colonel Milton S. Hall, a promoter and grading contractor who was commissioned by the Southern Pacific to grade the right-of-way between Spadra and Indio, built a very steep wagon road— known as Hall's Grade—up the mountainside from "Hall City" (near today's Cabezon) to a point above the present Lake Fulmor. Here he had a man named Fuller set up a small sawmill. Shortly afterward, Fuller moved the sawmill over the ridge and down to a new site above the present Fuller Mill Creek. The enterprise was none too successful. For one thing, the road was too precipitous for heavy loads, and at least two men were killed and several teams and loaded wagons smashed when they broke loose on the grade. After a frustrating year, the road was abandoned and the sawmill machinery hauled piece by piece down into lower Snow Creek Canyon. Here, at the bottom end of a dizzy skidway, it was set up to await the logs that never reached it. They either jumped the track or broke into splinters in their mad

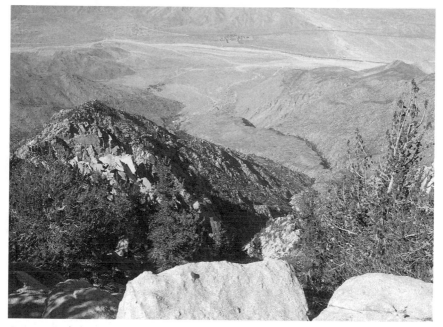

Snow Creek from San Jacinto Peak

rush from high on the mountain. By 1877 the Southern Pacific had its railroad through the pass and the costly logging efforts were abandoned. But Hall's Grade remained, later to become the springboard for other road-making projects in the mountains.

Much more successful were the logging enterprises on the west slope of the San Jacintos. In 1875, Joseph Crawford, Union Army veteran and homesteader at Oak Cliff in the San Jacinto Valley, secured a 50-year franchise from the San Diego County Board of Supervisors (San Diego County included the San Jacintos until 1893) to build a toll road from Oak Cliff up the west side of the mountains to Alvin Meadow and Strawberry Valley. Crawford spent $5,500 building his road into the timber belt, and even before it was finished loggers swarmed into the mountains. The road was narrow and just about as precipitous as Hall's Grade, and it elicited comments such as, "Steep? Why in places it leans over backwards!" There was a welcome water stop at Halfway House Spring, where teamsters and animals often collapsed.

Shortly after Crawford finished his toll road, large-scale logging efforts began on the western slopes. A number of sawmills were built along the North Fork of the San Jacinto River, in the vicinity of Dutch Flat, and in Strawberry Valley. Who built the first mill is not known for certain. Bradley and Stafford are believed to have erected the pioneer sawmill in Strawberry

Valley, then sold out around 1881 to Amasa Saunders, who built a spectacular overhead flume leading to a large waterwheel to operate his saws.
Saunders Meadow near Idyllwild honors him today. Anton Scherman had a
number of mills in and around Strawberry Valley, and at the peak of his operations was said to have cut 25,000 board feet per day. George B. Hannahs
purchased 4500 acres of timberland from the Southern Pacific Railroad[1] and
erected two mills—one at Dutch Flat, the other in Strawberry Valley. Hannah
is credited with starting the first settlement in Strawberry Valley, which he
named Raynetta after his infant son Raymond. His store was the focal point
for "outers, ranchers, cowboys, lumbermen, and everyone else attached to
the mountains by either business or pleasure." Here also was the first post
office in the San Jacinto Mountains, established in 1893. Hannahs was an
explorer too, and knew every foot of the mountains. He is credited with having named Round Valley and Long Valley and with discovering Hidden Lake,
which he called "Lake Surprise."

By the early 1890s, the timberlands of the western San Jacintos vibrated
to the thunder of falling trees, the swearing of tough woodsmen, the creak-
ing of wagons, and the whine of steel saws. Tall pines were cut from the
mountainside, hauled to mill by "bull teams," sliced into lumber, then wag-
oned down Crawford's toll road—the toll-keeper collected 75¢ per wag-
onload—to San Jacinto. Most of the lumber was sold and used in the San
Jacinto Valley; some was shipped to San Bernardino and Los Angeles.

Water-seekers came into the mountains, too. Ranchers in the San Jacinto
Valley needed water for their lands and saw in the San Jacinto Mountains a
ready source. In 1887, E.L. Mayberry, W.F. Whittier and other valley pioneers
formed the Lake Hemet Water Company to bring water down from the
mountains. A site was selected at the northwest end of Garner Valley, where
the South Fork of the San Jacinto River drops into a deep gorge. At the top
of this narrow canyon, a masonry dam was constructed. When the dam was
completed in 1893, it rose 122 feet above the canyon floor and formed a lake
of 600 acres. It was said to have been, at the time, the largest masonry dam
in the world. Water from the reservoir was carried to valley farms via a network of large wooden flumes.

Saving the San Jacintos

Acre by acre, the lumber monster was eating away at the mountain forest,
each year relentlessly cutting farther up the western slopes of the San
Jacintos. Sheep and cattle by the thousands were being herded to summer

---

1 In 1876 the Southern Pacific Railroad was given every other section of land for 11 miles on
both sides of their right-of-way, part of the federal government's huge subsidy program for
American big business during the later decades of the 19th century. Most of the San Jacinto
Mountains fell within this checkerboard pattern.

pasture in the high-country meadows, stripping them of their rich green cover. Wagon roads were being hacked higher and higher into the mountains. As with the San Gabriel and San Bernardino mountains, even those with myopic vision could see that reckless land-use practices were destroying both the beauty of the mountains and—more important to the practical-minded—the mountain watershed. Federal protection was called for. As a result of strong pressure from those who wanted the mountains saved, for either esthetic or practical reasons, President Grover Cleveland signed a bill creating the San Jacinto Forest Reserve on February 22, 1897. At first it was a forest reserve in name only, and not much was done to stop the continuing depredation. As with the San Bernardinos, much of the mountain lands were already in private hands—particularly the hands of the Southern Pacific Railroad—and outside Forest Service jurisdiction. In 1898 the first forest rangers were assigned to the reserve and a patrol system established. These early rangers of the old San Jacinto Forest Reserve—Charley Vandeventer, Theodore Olds, John Oloan, "Sulphur Springs" Thompson—did their job zealously, guarding against further timber cutting on public lands, chasing herders and their herds out of the high country, fighting brush fires, locating lost and injured persons. They set the standards followed by today's Forest Service in the San Jacintos. In 1907 the name was changed to San Jacinto National Forest, and the following year the San Jacinto was joined with the smaller Trabuco to create Cleveland National Forest. In 1925, the San Jacinto District was cut from the Cleveland and joined to San Bernardino National Forest. So it remains today.

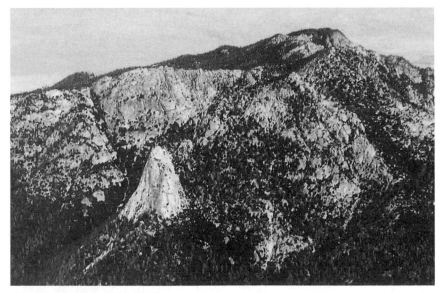

Tahquitz Peak and Lily Rock

Around the turn of the century, recreation replaced logging as the major activity in the San Jacinto Mountains. In 1893 or thereabouts, John and Mary Keen built their one-story Strawberry Valley Hotel, and a few years later started Keen Camp. In 1898 a group of Los Angeles doctors, headed by Dr. Walter Lindley and Dr. W.W. Becket, formed the California Health Resort Company and purchased 3500 acres in Strawberry Valley. Here they built a 3-story hotel and surrounding cottages for the treatment of tuberculosis patients. Around this sanitarium hotel a small resort community grew. In 1899 the federal government decided to relocate the post office in the hotel, at the time managed by Mrs. Laura Rutledge and her husband. Mrs. Rutledge suggested the name "Idyllwild" for the new post office and community. So it is known today. The first hotel, known as the Idyllwild Sanitarium, burned to the ground in 1904 and was replaced a few years later by the Idyllwild Inn, which became a popular summer resort. The Idyllwild Inn burned in 1945 and was replaced by the present structure. Through the years, particularly after World War II, Idyllwild has grown into a well-known resort community with a population today over 3000. It stands at the gateway to the San Jacinto Wilderness.

With the people came new roads. Crawford's old toll road was superseded in 1891 by the Mayberry Road, which followed basically today's State Highway 74 from the San Jacinto Valley to Keen Camp. Built by C.L. Mayberry, its original function was to transport materials for construction of Hemet Dam. From Keen Camp, Charley Thomas's old cattle trail to Strawberry Valley was improved into a road to Idyllwild. In 1909 the famous Idyllwild Control Road—one-way traffic only, alternating up and down every two hours—was constructed approximately along the route of Crawford's 1876 road. In 1911 the first primitive road from Banning to Idyllwild was constructed. In recent years, many of these roads have been improved and new ones built, allowing easy, high-gear access to the mountain communities.

Visiting the spectacular and beautiful San Jacinto high country—on foot or by horseback—has long been a favorite pastime of outdoor-minded Southern Californians. As early as 1885, parties camped in Round Valley and climbed to the top of San Jacinto Peak. After 1900, visits became much more frequent. Many of these early mountain visitors realized the need for safeguarding this unique alpine wilderness from the perils of unrestricted overuse and possible exploitation. First with a concrete proposal was A.C. Lovekin of Riverside, who in 1919 advocated setting aside the higher altitudes of the San Jacintos as a great wilderness memorial park in memory of those who gave their lives in World War I. Lovekin's plan met with general public approval, but nothing came of it for eight years. Then, in 1927, the California Legislature created the State Park System, and attention was once again focused on the Mount San Jacinto wilderness park proposal. In 1928

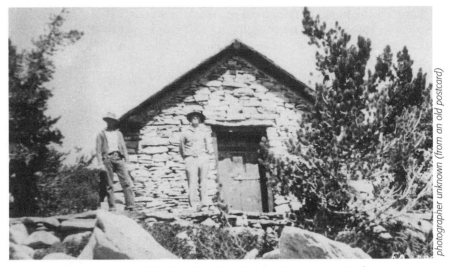

photographer unknown (from an old postcard)

Stone cabin built by the CCC in 1936, just below San Jacinto Peak

the San Jacinto State Park Association was formed, Lovekin as president, with the express purpose of including San Jacinto Peak and the surrounding high country in the State Park system. At the time, the main stumbling block was land ownership: the odd-numbered sections of land, including San Jacinto Peak itself, were owned by the Southern Pacific Company, while the even-numbered sections were federally owned lands administered by the Forest Service. The State Park Bond Act, passed by the California voters in 1928, and the pledge of matching funds from the Riverside County Board of Supervisors and private citizens, along with land purchase and exchange proposals acceptable to all involved parties, overcame this hurdle. In 1929 the State Park Commission formally adopted plans to acquire the lands and create Mount San Jacinto State Park, and by 1935 all the land atop the range was in state ownership. The valuation of the 12,695 acres within the park, acquired in a 3-way deal with the Southern Pacific Land Company, the U.S. Forest Service and the State of California, was $84,218.75. Half of this sum was contributed by Riverside County and friends of the park project. The federal government aided greatly in the development of the park through the Civilian Conservation Corps (CCC) program. In 1935–36, gangs of young CCC workers camped in Round Valley, Tahquitz Valley and near Idyllwild, built 26 miles of trail, developed 29 campsites, and erected the stone refuge cabin on San Jacinto Peak. June 19, 1937 was a memorable day to conservationists and lovers of the San Jacinto high country; Mount San Jacinto State Park was formally dedicated. Since then, parcels of land have been added, and in 1963 the name was expanded to Mount San Jacinto Wilderness State Park.

In 1931 the Forest Service designated the mountain regions immediately north and south of the state park as the San Jacinto Wild Area. In 1964 the name was changed to San Jacinto Wilderness. The entire top country of the range, from Fuller Ridge on the north side to the Desert Divide south of Tahquitz Peak is now protected by the state and federal wilderness systems.

Caught Off-guard

The story of the San Jacinto high country would end here if it were not for the determined efforts of two Palm Springs businessmen. In 1935 Francis F. Crocker of the California Electric Power Company and Carl Barkow of the Desert Sun newspaper presented the idea of a tramway (from Palm Springs up the north face of San Jacinto Mountain) to the Palm Springs Chamber of Commerce. The idea quickly caught on, particularly because it was felt that a spectacular mountain tramway would be a boon to the Palm Springs tourist industry. In 1939 a bill was introduced in the State Legislature to establish a "Palm Springs Winter Parks Authority" to build the tramway. It passed the legislature but was vetoed by Governor Olson. Similar bills, slightly changed, were introduced in 1941 and 1943, but both met the same fate. In 1945 a fourth bill was drawn up, this time with considerable change of language. The proposed agency was now called the "Mount San Jacinto Winter Park Authority" and benefits to all Californians, including skiers, were advertised. The appeal to skiers was a brazen smokescreen: the Far West Ski Association pointed out that, because of the craggy nature of the mountain, skiing here was highly unsuitable. But conservationists were caught with their guard down, and the bill sailed through the legislature and was signed by Governor Warren. The undisguised purpose of the Winter Park Authority was to build a tramway up the north wall of the mountain for the benefit of Palm Springs, and it quickly set about to achieve this goal. But it was a long time reaching it.

For the next 15 years—until actual construction began in 1961—one of the most bitter battles between conservationists and business developers ever fought in California raged over the tramway proposal. Charges and counter-charges flew back and forth, and both sides used every weapon in their legal arsenal to advance or defeat the project. A residue of bitterness remains to this day. Finally the last legal obstruction was batted down, $7,700,000 in revenue bonds to finance construction were sold, construction was commenced, and the spectacular aerial tramway became a reality in 1963. The Mount San Jacinto Winter Park Authority threw off any vestige of disguise for its true motive when it named the completed project the "Palm Springs Aerial Tramway." From Valley Station in Chino Canyon at an elevation of 2643', two gondolas suspended on wires supported by five towers whisk visitors over a mile in elevation gain to Mountain Station, located at 8516' on the edge of Long Valley. It is a steep and breathtaking rise for the

80 passengers on each gondola. And it gives almost instant access to a part of the high wilderness that once required several hours of strenuous hiking to reach. Such is the form of "progress."

The San Jacinto high country is a priceless heirloom of the people of Southern California. Sheer numbers of visitors, increasing every year, constitute what is perhaps the biggest threat to the wilderness character of the mountains. (Unless you take seriously the hare-brained schemes, voiced now and then, to build an extension of the tramway to the top of San Jacinto Peak.) To counter the weight of numbers, the state and the U.S. Forest Service instituted the wilderness permit system in 1971, which developed the present quotas for overnight use. Only with wisdom and restraint will Southern California's best mountain wilderness be preserved.

Just below the high country, battles are being fought too. In a landmark citizen-action campaign in the 1970s, the San Jacinto Mountain Conservation League (Box 1872, Hemet, CA 92343) defeated a developer's proposal to urbanize Garner Valley before a land-use plan and zoning regulations were worked out. With zoning now accomplished, the league's next aim is to get the valley preserved as national forest through federal land exchanges. Some land exchanges have been made, but much remains to be done.

In recent years, development has crept forward in Garner Valley and around the fringes of the San Jacinto Wilderness and State Park. But fortunately, the high country has remained inviolate, and the desert side of the mountains is now protected by the Santa Rosa and San Jacinto Mountains National Monument, established by Congress in 2000. The future of the San Jacinto Mountains requires constant vigilance.

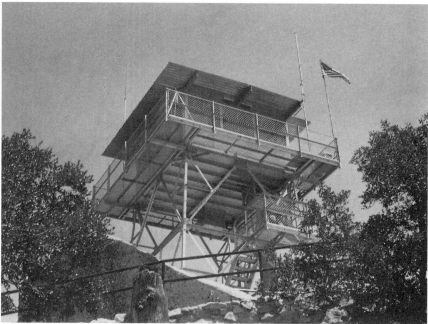

Black Mountain Lookout (Hike 57)

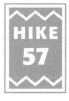

BLACK MOUNTAIN

Hike Length: 7 miles round trip; 2600' elevation gain
Difficulty: Moderate
Season: All year
Topo map: *Lake Fulmor* (7.5'),
San Jacinto Wilderness (Tom Harrison)

Features

Black Mountain at 7772 feet dominates the northern end of the San Jacintos. From the fire lookout, you are rewarded with a superb vista over miles of mountain, valley and desert country, with the jagged ramparts of San Jacinto Peak looming in the southeast.

Description

From Banning drive southeast on State Highway 243 1.0 mile beyond Vista Grande Ranger Station to the beginning of the Black Mountain Trail (2E35) marked by a large wooden sign at mile marker 243 RIV 16.75. Turn left and drive 100 yards on a dirt road to the parking area (**GPS SB57**).

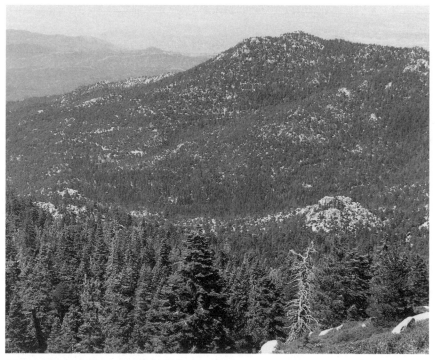

Black Mountain from Forsee Ridge

Proceed up the trail through charred remains of Jeffrey pine, oak and chaparral. The trail climbs 2.5 miles up the ridge, passing through the heart of the burned forest, crosses a divide, leaves the burned area, and contours into a shady forest to Indian Creek (water in spring only). You then climb steeply up to a pine-shaded flat on the ridgetop known as Shake Camp (no overnight camping) and switchback up the forested slope to a spur of the Black Mountain lookout road, 3.5 miles out. Turn right and walk the short distance to the summit lookout tower.

Return the same way. An option, with a 9-mile car shuttle, is to descend the lookout road (4S68), passing Boulder Basin Public Campground, to Black Mountain Road (4S01), 1 mile. To reach this junction, drive up State Highway 243, passing Lake Fulmor, to Black Mountain Road, 4.2 miles from the Black Mountain trailhead. Turn left (north) and drive up Black Mountain Road to its junction with the side road to Boulder Basin Campground, 4.8 miles. Park here (**GPS SB57A**), or pay the campground fee at Boulder Basin, 0.4 mile farther (**GPS SB57B**).

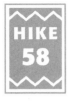

SAN JACINTO PEAK VIA FULLER RIDGE TRAIL

Hike Length: 15 miles round trip; 4100' elevation gain
Difficulty: Strenuous (1 day), Moderate (2 days)
Season: June–October
Topo maps: *Lake Fulmor, San Jacinto Peak* (both 7.5'), *San Jacinto Wilderness* (Tom Harrison)
Permit: San Jacinto Wilderness Permit required

Features

From Black Mountain, the craggy spine of Fuller Ridge dips downward and then soars upward, like a long kite string, to Folly Peak. Broken gendarmes and huge granite outcroppings make it one of the most rugged mountain backbones in Southern California. Weather-toughened pines and firs cling to its precipitous slopes.

The Fuller Ridge Trail threads its way around these gray-white gendarmes, first on the north side of the ridge, then on the south, from the Black Mountain Road to the Deer Springs Trail below San Jacinto Peak. Views are magnificent, particularly down into the wild and beautiful gorge of upper Snow Creek and beyond to the desert. Much less traveled than the heavily used trails out of Idyllwild and the Palm Springs Aerial Tramway, this ranks as one of the best trips in the San Jacintos.

This trip takes the Fuller Ridge Trail to Deer Springs, then uses the Deer Springs Trail to ascend San Jacinto Peak (10,804'). You can do it in one very long day, or make it more leisurely by staying the night at Little Round Valley Trail Camp. (*Note:* Deer Springs Trail Camp and the summit camping area have been closed because of overuse.)

Although the summit is only 3100' above the trailhead, the trail dips and climbs several times to bypass rock obstacles on the ridge, adding a bonus 500' of elevation on the ascent, then again on the weary descent.

Description

From State Highway 243 1.3 miles southeast of the Indian Vista turnout and 0.5 mile east of mile marker 243 RIV 13.00, turn northeast up the good dirt Black Mountain Road. After 4.8 miles, pass a side road on your left to Black Mountain Campground and fire lookout. Your road winds through spectacular open forest with giant granite boulders. It passes the entrance of the Black Mountain Group Camp after 1.0 mile, then a rocky outcropping on the left in another 0.8 mile featuring spectacular views of San Gorgonio Mountain and the pass below. In another 0.7 mile, turn right up a hill at a sign for the Fuller Ridge Trailhead. Climb 0.2 mile and park in the clearing (**GPS SB58**).

The trail, which is a segment of the Pacific Crest Trail, rounds the north side of the slope and climbs through pine, cedar, and fir to a notch in Fuller Ridge, 2 miles. Along the way, you will find gooseberries and huge bushes of red and blue currants. You then drop, climb, and contour around granite outcroppings on both sides of the ridge, with spectacular views through "windows" in the rocky spine. You can peer down into the extremely rugged upper reaches of Snow Creek's west fork, where there are the remains of the flume in which Colonel Hall tried to drop timber from the mountain forest to the desert in 1876. Southward, you look down into the forested bowl of Fuller Mill Creek, once the scene of large-scale logging. After another mile you begin to contour, then climb along the southwest slope of the San Jacinto massif, passing two small creeks of icy-cold water, to a junction with the Deer Springs Trail, 5 miles from the start.

Go left (northeast) up the slope, and follow the Deer Springs Trail past small Boggy Meadow to Little Round Valley Trail Camp, 1 mile above the junction (see Hike 66 for a full description of the Deer Springs Trail). You are in lodgepole forest now. From Little Round Valley, continue up the trail to a junction with the San Jacinto Peak Trail, 1.25 miles. Turn left and climb past the stone shelter cabin to the summit, 300 yards. Camping is not allowed on the peak.

Return the same way—or, with a car shuttle, take one of the numerous options that are open to you (see Hikes 61, 62, 66, 68). Alternatively, climbers can cross-country over to Folly Peak, then down the brush-spotted ridge to the Fuller Ridge/Pacific Crest Trail halfway between the Deer Springs Trail junction and the roadhead, but don't attempt this unless you are experienced in cross-country travel. Rock hopping along the crest of the ridge can be fun and keeps you clear of the worst of the brush until the last 400', where wading through chinquapin and brushing aside sappy trees becomes inevitable. The final 100 yards cross a flat of dense chaparral to pick up the PCT just left of a rocky outcrop at 8700'.

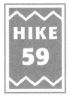

INDIAN MOUNTAIN

HIKE 59

Hike Length: 5 miles round trip; 800' elevation gain
Difficulty: Easy
Season: November–June
(fire closure 7/1 to winter rain)
Topo map: *Lake Fulmor* (7.5'),
San Jacinto Wilderness (Tom Harrison)

Features

Indian Mountain rises to 5790 feet over the western foothills of the range, offering a splendid panorama over chaparral-coated hillsides and the flat expanse of San Jacinto Valley. This trip is a fire-road walk most of the way, best done on a cool, clear winter or spring day.

The south slopes of Indian Mountain were blackened by the 1997 Bee Canyon fire, but fortunately the chaparral is quickly growing back tall and verdant.

Description

From Banning, drive southeast on State Highway 243 to the Indian Vista overlook parking area 0.6 mile past the Lake Fulmer picnic area and just past mileage marker 243 RIV 14.00 (**GPS SB59**). The Indian Mountain fire road (4S21) begins just northwest of the overlook parking area.

Walk through the gate (usually open for recreational vehicles) and down the fire road to a saddle, then up and around the east and south slopes of Indian Mountain—mostly through chaparral country, with clumps of Jeffrey pine and oak offering occasional shade. The fire road climbs almost to the summit on the south side before beginning its 6-mile descent to State Highway 74. When it reaches its high point, turn right and follow the old, partly overgrown firebreak to the boulder-strewn summit.

Return the same way.

NORTH FORK, SAN JACINTO RIVER

HIKE
60

Hike Length: 1–4 miles round trip; 200' elevation gain
Difficulty: Easy to moderate
Season: May–October
Topo map: *San Jacinto Peak* (7.5'),
San Jacinto Wilderness (Tom Harrison)

Features

There is no better place to experience the riparian delights of the San Jacintos than along the North Fork of the San Jacinto River. The musical waters of the creek exhibit a delightful variety of moods—now splashing merrily over boulders, now pausing in limpid pools, only to plunge headlong over miniature waterfalls and cascades. Along its banks sprout western azalea, its sweet-smelling gold and white flowers often growing under western dogwood, splendid in spring with flower-like clusters of white bracts and just as glorious in fall when its leaves turn burgundy-red. Scarlet monkeyflower and pale columbine cheer these shady thickets with colorful blooms, all under a verdant canopy of alder, willow, and bay. On the slopes above is a mixed forest of live oak, incense-cedar, ponderosa and Jeffrey pine, all contributing to nature's soft picture of elegance.

This trip is more of a saunter than a hike, a place to contemplate the gifts of the natural world and briefly forget civilization's tribulations. You can go as far as you want—a few hundred yards beside the dancing waters, or a mile or more over and around the streamside boulders into hidden recesses.

The area is of special biological interest as well since it is one of the last remaining populated habitats in the San Bernardino National Forest for the federally endangered Mountain Yellow-Legged Frog. This frog was historically one of the most common frogs in Southern California and used to be found in virtually every year-round stream in the mountains, but has declined in 99% of its range in the last couple decades. Due to the presence of this sensitive species and others, the Forest Service asks visitors to avoid wading, rock hopping, fishing, and other water play within 10 feet of the creek edge. Watch for posted signs in the area with the latest information or check with the Idyllwild Ranger Station.

Description

From Banning, drive southeast on State Highway 243 to its crossing of the signed North Fork of the San Jacinto River at mile marker 243 RIV 11.25, 0.7 mile past Fuller Mill Creek picnic area (**GPS SB60**). There is a large parking area on the south side of the highway about 50 yards west of the North Fork crossing and a small parking area on the north side adjacent to the creek.

Just west of the highway bridge, on the north side, follow a use trail that drops steeply down to the creek. The trail forks often with most side paths leading down toward the stream, but there is a main use path that continues weaving around boulders and logs along the southeast side of the creek and once crossing a small tributary. Farther up, there are a few places where you must scramble to get around rock obstructions. If you are a beginner, a half mile is about as far as you should go. It is possible to follow the North Fork all the way up to Dark Canyon Public Campground, but this is for experienced hikers only as slopes near the end become steep and slippery. Once at the campground, the creek flows under a bridge and the use trails continue along the northwest side of the creek up to the State Wilderness boundary and Seven Pines Trail crossing. Wear boots with good tread and ankle support.

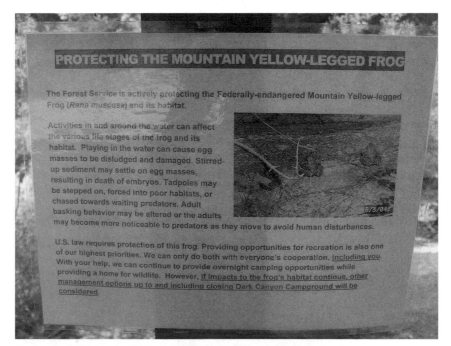

Endanged Mountain Yellow-Legged Frog (*Rana muscose*)

DEER SPRINGS

HIKE 61

Hike Length: 7.5 miles round trip; 2600' elevation gain
Difficulty: Moderate
Season: June–October
Topo maps: *San Jacinto Peak* (7.5'),
San Jacinto Wilderness (Tom Harrison)
Permit: San Jacinto Wilderness Permit required

Features

The Seven Pines Trail climbs the ridge between Fuller Mill Creek and Dark Canyon and continues up to Deer Springs. You wind through granite outcroppings and beautiful forest country, with views now and then toward the rugged headwall of Fuller Ridge. It is a steep but pleasant walk on a good trail, crossing and recrossing the tumbling North Fork, with several options for the return.

Description

Drive 200 yards east of Alandale Ranger Station on State Highway 243 (near mile marker 243 RIV 9.75, 19 miles from Banning, 6 miles from Idyllwild), then up the paved Marion Mtn. Road (4S02), going left at a junction in 100 yards and left again in 0.8 mile, to Dark Canyon Public Campground. Follow the one-way loop road right through the campground to rejoin 4S02 as a fair dirt road just past the top of the loop. Turn right and follow 4S02, passing Azalea Trails Girl Scout Camp, to the signed Seven Pines 2E13 trailhead, on your right, 4.3 miles out (**GPS SB61**).

Follow the trail as it climbs up the boulder-stacked, forested ridge between Fuller Mill Creek and Dark Canyon. In 1.25 miles you cross the ridgecrest and drop to the North Fork, where you enter San Jacinto State Park Wilderness. The trail fords the creek and climbs east, crossing and recrossing the North Fork, to a junction with Deer Springs Trail, 3.5 miles from the start. Turn left (east) and follow the latter to Deer Springs, 0.25 mile. There is water here but overnight camping is not allowed.

Return the way you came. Options are to descend the Marion Mountain Trail (Hike 62), the Deer Springs Trail to Idyllwild (Hike 66), or the Fuller Ridge Trail to Black Mountain Road (Hike 58). All require car shuttles.

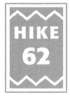

SAN JACINTO PEAK
VIA MARION MOUNTAIN TRAIL

Hike Length: 12 miles round trip; 4600' elevation gain
Difficulty: Strenuous (1 day), Moderate (2 days)
Season: June–October
Topo map: *San Jacinto Peak* (7.5'),
San Jacinto Wilderness (Tom Harrison)
Permit: San Jacinto Wilderness Permit required

Features

This is the shortest way to climb San Jacinto Peak from the southwest slope; it is also very steep in places. Old-timers call this a no-nonsense route—right up the mountainside in short, steep zigzags. The first 2.25 miles are the most strenuous; you gain 2200' from the new trailhead just below Marion Mountain Campground to Deer Springs. The remainder of the route is only slightly less precipitous—2400' more gain in 3.25 miles via the Deer Springs Trail. You can do it in one exhausting pull, or make it more enjoyable by spending the night at Little Round Valley Trail Camp. This trip is a living demonstration of forest change with altitude—you start up in Jeffrey pine and oak, climb through a belt of sugar pine and white fir, then into lodgepole pine interspersed with thickets of manzanita, snow brush, and chinquapin, and finally emerge above timberline at the summit.

Description

From 200 yards east of Alandale Ranger Station on State Highway 243 (near mile marker 243 RIV 9.75, 19 miles from Banning or 6 miles from Idyllwild), drive up the paved Marion Mtn. Road (4S02), going left at a junction in 100 yards, to a junction with Marion Mountain Campground Road (4S71) in 0.8 mile. Go right and follow the latter for 0.6 mile, passing the entrance to Fern Basin Campground, to the Marion Mountain trailhead (**GPS SB62**), just short of Marion Mountain Campground. The parking area on your left has space for 10 to 12 vehicles.

Cross 4S71 to the signed MARION MOUNTAIN TRAIL (2E14). You climb through pines and cedars, passing a short access trail coming up from Marion Mountain Campground, then ascend steeply up the northwest flank of forested Marion Ridge to a junction with the Deer Springs Trail, 2.25 miles. Turn left and follow the latter footpath 0.25 mile to Deer Springs. Water is available here but no camping. Continue up the Deer Springs Trail past Boggy Meadows to Little Round Valley Trail Camp, nestled snugly in a small, sandy basin just below the peak. Water is available here through late summer but should be purified before drinking. Continue up the trail to a junction with the short San Jacinto Peak Trail, 1 mile. Turn left and climb the latter, passing the stone shelter cabin built by the CCC in 1936, to the 10,804' summit, less than 0.25 mile. Camping is not allowed in the summit area.

Return the same way. Another way down, requiring a 3-mile car shuttle, is via the Seven Pines Trail (Hike 61). With much longer car shuttles, you can descend the Fuller Ridge/Pacific Crest Trail to Black Mountain Road (Hike 58), the Deer Springs Trail to Idyllwild (Hike 66), the Wellman Cienega Trail to Humber Park (Hike 68), or, with a very lengthy car shuttle, via Round and Long valleys to the Palm Springs Aerial Tramway (Hike 85).

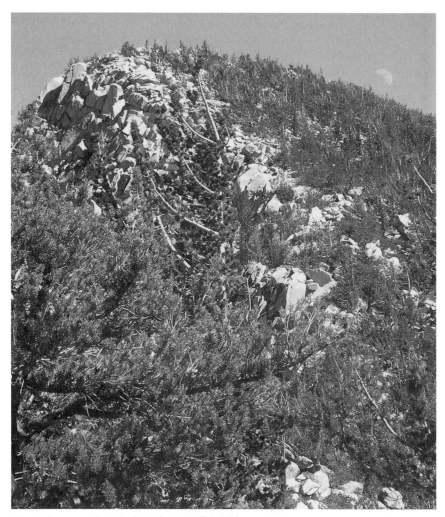

Moonrise over San Jacinto from Fuller Ridge

WEBSTER TRAIL

Hike Length: 5 miles round trip;
1900′ elevation loss and gain
Difficulty: Moderate
Season: October–June
Topo map: *Lake Fulmor, San Jacinto Peak* (both 7.5′),
San Jacinto Wilderness (Tom Harrison)

Features

The North Fork of the San Jacinto River cuts a deep swath down the west slope of the range. Melting snows and gushing springs high on the western ramparts of San Jacinto Peak nourish the several streams that join to become the North Fork; then the united waters tumble down the broad, V-shaped chasm to join with the South Fork, just above the San Jacinto Valley. A green canopy of fir, pine, cedar, and oak shades the stream for most of its length. This trip drops into the lonely middle reaches of the North Fork via the old Webster Trail, named for David G. Webster, pioneer rancher at Valle Vista in the San Jacinto Valley, who drove cattle up to high pasture on this path in the 1870s and '80s. Helen Hunt Jackson patterned her character Merrill in *Ramona* after Webster, whom she met while researching conditions of Native Americans in the San Jacinto Valley.

This is an ideal outing for a cool winter or spring day. You start under Jeffrey pines and live oaks, drop down slopes covered with chaparral, swiftly growing back after a fire, and reach a secluded part of the creek, spotted with tall pines, oaks, and alders. Try it after a rain, when the streams run full and the aroma of damp chaparral perfumes the air. Allow plenty of time for the return trip—it's all uphill.

Description

From Pine Cove at the Shell station on State Highway 243, 3 miles from Idyllwild and just north of mile marker 247 RIV 7.25, turn west on Pine Cove Road and follow it for 0.8 mile as it curves north to a junction with Forest Roads 5S09 and 5S10. Turn sharp left (southwest) on 5S10 and continue to a junction at the Lia Hona Lodge. Turn right and descend 0.9 mile on a fair dirt road to the beginning of the Webster Trail, indicated by a wooden sign on the right. Park in the adjacent clearing (**GPS SB63**).

Follow the trail west as it descends the ridge, first through an open forest of Jeffrey pine and oak, then through dense chaparral. Your view is superb if the day is clear—across velvet-coated foothills to the flat expanse of the San Jacinto Valley. The dirt road you see climbing the next ridge south is part of the old Hemet-Idyllwild control road, used from 1910 to 1929, one-way traffic only. Where the slope begins to descend more steeply as it nears the gorge, the trail makes one long switchback south and reaches the cool waters of the North Fork, 2.5 miles from the start.

After your streamside rest amid sylvan greenery, return the way you came—all uphill now.

SUICIDE ROCK

HIKE 64

Hike Length: 7 miles round trip; 1900' elevation gain
Difficulty: Moderate
Season: May–October
Topo map: *San Jacinto Peak* (7.5'),
San Jacinto Wilderness (Tom Harrison)
Permit: San Jacinto Wilderness Permit required

Features

Suicide Rock (7528') is an outcropping of white granite that juts from the south slope of Marion Ridge, high above Strawberry Valley. Legend says that Suicide Rock was so named after a Native American maiden and her lover jumped to their deaths from its rim rather than live without each other as had been decreed by the tribal chief. A splendid panorama of the valley floor covered with dense forest, the village of Idyllwild, and the rugged granite cliffs of Lily Rock and Tahquitz Peak awaits the hiker who reaches this viewpoint. This relatively short trip takes the Deer Springs Trail to Suicide Junction, then a side trail over to the rock.

Description

From Idyllwild Ranger Station drive west 1 mile on the Banning–Idyllwild Highway (State Highway 243). Park on the north side of the road just above the County Park Nature Center and past a sign pointing to Deer Springs Trailhead Parking (**GPS SB64**). The Deer Springs Trail itself (3E17) starts 50 yards down the road. Alternatively, walk up a steep unmarked path above the parking area for 150 yards to a junction with the Deer Springs Trail near some power lines. Turn left and proceed uphill.

Your trail follows an abandoned dirt road about 200 yards, then turns right (north) and climbs steadily through an open forest of oak, Jeffrey pine, and king-sized manzanita to the ridgetop. You switchback up the ridge to a signed junction with the Suicide Rock Trail, 2.3 miles from the start. Here you leave the Deer Springs Trail and turn east, following the lateral trail as it contours across slopes clothed with pine and fir, crosses the trickle of Marion Creek, and climbs the back side of Suicide Rock to the abrupt rim overlooking Strawberry Valley, 1 mile from the junction. The white dome you see directly across the valley is Lily Rock; the steepled granite summit on the skyline is Tahquitz Peak.

Return the same way.

STRAWBERRY-SADDLE LOOP

HIKE 65

Hike Length:	11 miles round trip; 3100' elevation gain
Difficulty:	Moderate
Season:	June–October
Topo map:	*San Jacinto Peak* (7.5'),
	San Jacinto Wilderness (Tom Harrison)
Permit:	San Jacinto Wilderness Permit required

Features

Although bordered by desert and semi-arid hill country, the San Jacintos are a particularly lush mountain range. Nowhere is this more evident than at the numerous springs and marshy cienagas that dot the upper slopes. The abundant rain and snow that fall at the high elevations seep into the porous granite, which acts as a natural storage reservoir. Water from this rock reservoir flows out at many points high in the mountains, forming emerald-green and flowery marshes threaded by clear, gurgling streamlets. One of the lushest of these sloping mountainside gardens is Strawberry Cienaga, high on the south face of Marion Mountain.

This loop trip—requiring a short car shuttle between Idyllwild and Humber Park—climbs the Deer Springs Trail to Strawberry Junction, contours across the steep south slope of Marion Mountain to Strawberry Cienaga, then descends the Wellman Trail to Saddle Junction and the Devils Slide to Humber Park. It is a delightful daylong hike on good trail all the way, passing through rich forest and meadow country, with continuous views of the Yosemite-like cliffs and ridges of Tahquitz Peak and Lily Rock.

Description

From Idyllwild Ranger Station drive west 1 mile on the Banning–Idyllwild Highway (State Highway 243). Park on the north side of the road just above the County Park Nature Center and past a sign pointing to Deer Springs Trailhead Parking (**GPS SB64**). The Deer Springs Trail itself (3E17) starts 50 yards down the road. Leave another vehicle at Humber Park: From Highway 243 in Idyllwild just below the ranger station, turn northeast on North Circle Dr. Drive 0.7 mile to a four way intersection, then turn right on South Circle Dr. Proceed 0.1 mile, then turn left on Fern Valley Road. After 1.7 miles, reach a small parking area for the Ernie Maxwell Scenic Trail. Continue 0.1 mile up the hill to the outhouse and larger parking area of Humber Park (**GPS SB67**).

Follow the Deer Springs Trail as it climbs northward to a junction with the Strawberry Cienaga Trail, 4.1 miles from the start (1.8 miles beyond the Suicide Rock Trail junction). Turn right (east) and follow the Strawberry

Cienaga lateral trail across the south face of Marion Mountain, through open stands of lodgepole pine and white fir, to Strawberry Cienaga. There is no overnight camping here, but there are nice picnic spots alongside clear, cold rivulets. Your view across the valley to the rugged spurs of Tahquitz Peak is breathtaking.

Continue east along the trail to a junction with the Wellman Cienaga Trail, 2.3 miles from the Deer Springs Trail. Turn right (south) and descend the boulder-stacked ridge, through scattered Jeffrey pines, to the 5-way Saddle Junction, 1.9 miles. Turn right again (west) and descend the Devils Slide Trail to Humber Park, 2.5 miles (see Hike 67 for full description).

An easier option, with 700 feet less elevation gain, is to do the trip in reverse, starting at Humber Park and ending at Deer Springs trailhead.

Another option is to start or end the hike at the Suicide Rock climbers trail rather than Deer Springs, avoiding the car shuttle. The climbers trail begins at a small maker 1.4 miles up Fern Valley Road and 0.4 mile below Humber Park (**GPS SB65A**). The trail reaches the top of Suicide Rock, where it joins a path to the Deer Springs Trail (see Hike 64). This trail passes through private property with permission of the owners. Please respect their land and do not stray from the trail.

SAN JACINTO PEAK FROM IDYLLWILD

HIKE 66

Hike Length: 19 miles round trip; 5200' elevation gain
Difficulty: Very Strenuous (1 day), Moderate (2 days)
Season: June–October
Topo map: *San Jacinto Peak* (7.5'),
San Jacinto Wilderness (Tom Harrison)
Permit: San Jacinto Wilderness Permit required

Features

The western slopes of San Jacinto Peak and the long, sinuous ridge of Marion Mountain are blanketed with dense stands of pine, fir, and cedar, interspaced here and there with manzanita and chinquapin thickets and, where water seeps to the surface, verdant meadows. The Deer Springs Trail, a popular hikers' route built by the CCC during the 1930s, threads most of the length of this slope, then climbs steeply to within a stone's throw of the summit.

This trip makes use of the Deer Springs Trail to ascend San Jacinto Peak, then loops around and back through Wellman and Strawberry cienagas on the return. Enroute you pass two trail camps—Strawberry Junction, 3 miles up the trail where the Strawberry Cienaga Trail meets your route, and Little Round Valley, high on a lodgepole-pine-shaded bench under San Jacinto Peak. There is water at Little Round Valley until late summer, but it should be purified before drinking. Choose one for your overnight stay; the next day, climb to the summit for a panorama unsurpassed in Southern California, and circle back via the two cienagas.

Description

From Idyllwild Ranger Station drive west 1 mile on the Banning–Idyllwild Highway (State Highway 243). Park on the north side of the road just above the County Park Nature Center and past a sign pointing to Deer Springs Trailhead Parking (**GPS SB64**). The Deer Springs Trail itself (3E17) starts 50 yards down the road. Alternatively, walk up a steep unmarked path above the parking area for 150 yards to a junction with the Deer Springs Trail near some power lines.

Proceed northward up the Deer Springs Trail, through alternate stands of oak, Jeffrey pine, and manzanita, passing junctions with the Suicide Rock and Strawberry Cienaga trails, to the top of Marion Ridge, 5 miles. Your path now contours and climbs through a dense forest of pine and fir and crosses several trickling streamlets of icy-cold water. You pass junctions with the Marion Mountain Trail (Hike 62) and the Seven Pines Trail (Hike 61), both leading down to your left, and continue to Deer Springs, 6.4 miles from the start. There is water here but the trail camp has been closed because of severe overuse. From Deer Springs, the trail climbs 200 yards to a junction with the Fuller Ridge/Pacific Crest Trail (Hike 58). Go right (northeast), up a steep slope covered with manzanita, snow brush and chinquapin, across a marshy bench known as Boggy Meadows, and up to Little Round Valley, 1.5 miles from Deer Springs. Here also are plentiful campsites amid lodgepole pine under granite spurs. You'll find water here until late summer, but you should purify it before drinking. From Little Round Valley, the trail climbs steeply through lodgepoles to a junction with the San Jacinto Peak Trail, 1.3 miles. Turn left and climb past the stone shelter building to the boulder-stacked summit, 300 yards.

After taking in the fabulous view, return to the before-mentioned junction. Turn left (southeast) and descend the main trail (see Hike 68 for a full description) past Wellman Divide and Wellman Cienaga to a junction with the Strawberry Cienaga Lateral Trail, 3 miles. Turn right (west) on the latter and follow it 2.25 miles through Strawberry Cienaga (see Hike 65) to its junction with the Deer Springs Trail. Strawberry Junction Trail Camp is here, with water available from Stone Creek about 100 yards up the Deer Springs Trail. Turn left (south) and descend the Deer Springs Trail to Idyllwild.

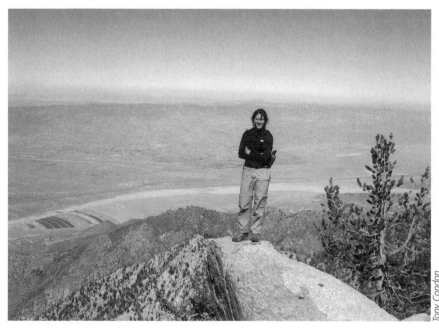

The summit of San Jacinto

SKUNK CABBAGE MEADOW

HIKE 67

Hike Length: 6 miles round trip; 1600' elevation gain
Difficulty: Moderate
Season: June–October
Topo maps: *San Jacinto Peak* (7.5'),
San Jacinto Wilderness (Tom Harrison)
Permit: San Jacinto Wilderness Permit required

Features

The Devils Slide Trail is the hikers' main gateway into the San Jacinto Wilderness. The trail climbs the steep mountain wall above the head of Strawberry Valley in long, easy-graded switchbacks, then abruptly crosses the crest to Saddle Junction, the takeoff point for footpaths leading in five directions. En route you pass through beautiful stands of oak, pine, cedar, and fir, with patches of manzanita and snow brush just below the top. Three trickling rills—Jolley Spring, Middle Spring and Powderbox Spring—offer trailside refreshment in early season, but dry up one by one as summer fades into fall.

The Devils Slide Trail today is a gradual uphill climb, certainly undeserving of its notorious name. But once it was quite different. In pioneer days, when Charley Thomas and later Frank Wellman drove cattle up the mountain to feed on the rich grasses of Tahquitz Valley, it was a frightful climb. No switchbacks then, just right up the mountainside, over loose boulders and fallen trees, through thorny chaparral thickets. Many a cow and even a few cowboys took a neck-breaking spill on this treacherous slope, and anyone who knew the Devils Slide then always remembered it. Since then, the Devils Slide Trail has been worked and reworked many times, until it in no way resembles its historical namesake. In fact, it has become so gentle that one wiseacre has suggested the name be changed to "Angels' Walk."

This rather short trip uses the Devils Slide Trail to offer a small sampling of the beautiful San Jacinto Wilderness. You climb to Saddle Junction, then continue a slight distance to Skunk Cabbage Meadow, an emerald-green oasis set amid the dark forest. Here is Skunk Cabbage Trail Camp, with spring water, stoves, and toilet. An overnight stay here is guaranteed to please.

Description

From Highway 243 in Idyllwild just below the ranger station, turn northeast on North Circle Dr. Drive 0.7 mile, passing Nomad Ventures (a good outdoors and climbing shop). At the 4-way intersection, turn right on South Circle Dr. Proceed 0.1 mile, then turn left on Fern Valley Road. After 1.7

miles, reach a small parking area for the Ernie Maxwell Scenic Trail. Continue 0.1 mile up the hill to the outhouse and larger parking area of Humber Park (**GPS SB67**).

The Devils Slide Trail starts from the top of the parking area, under the shadow of towering Lily Rock. You zigzag up the mountainside through a varied forest of Jeffrey pine, incense-cedar, white fir, and several species of oak. As you gain elevation, the views south over Strawberry Valley and north across the canyon to the precipitous south slope of Marion Mountain become impressive. In 1.25 miles, a small rivulet coming down from Jolley Spring is passed. The trail then makes a long switchback out across oak- and manzanita-covered slopes and passes minute Middle Spring. The trail then re-enters the pine and fir forest, passes Powderbox Spring, and crosses a low point in the rim to Saddle Junction, 2.5 miles. Here, on the heavily-forested tableland, is a 5-way trail fork (see Hikes 68, 70, 72 and 73 for particulars). A sign points to the northeast fork as leading to Skunk Cabbage Meadow. Proceed this way, through a lush forest of tall Jeffrey pines with ferns matting the floor, to another junction, 0.5 mile. Turn right (south) as indicated by the sign and walk 0.25 mile farther to the verdant clearing of Skunk Cabbage Meadow. (*Note:* take particular care here on this part of the table-land—trails criss-cross in all directions. Fortunately most of them are well marked.)

From Skunk Cabbage Meadow, short exploratory trips are possible to Willow Creek (see Hike 70), Tahquitz Valley and Tahquitz Creek (see Hike 71). Longer side trips are possible to points too numerous to mention here (see Hikes 68, 72 and 73). Because of its central location, Skunk Cabbage makes an ideal campsite.

Return the way you came.

SAN JACINTO PEAK FROM HUMBER PARK

HIKE 68

Hike Length:	16 miles round trip; 4400' elevation gain
Difficulty:	Moderate (2 days), Strenuous (1 day)
Season:	June–October
Topo map:	*San Jacinto Peak* (7.5'),
	San Jacinto Wilderness (Tom Harrison)
Permit:	San Jacinto Wilderness Permit required

Features

When naturalist John Muir stood on the summit and watched the sunrise in 1896, he is said to have exclaimed: "The view from San Jacinto is the most sublime spectacle to be found anywhere on this earth!"[1] Since then, countless others have experienced Muir's inspiration. The vista is utterly magnificent, extending over hundreds of square miles of mountains, foothills, valleys, and desert. On the western horizon, beyond row after row of misty-purple ranges, is the glimmering Pacific. Northwest, the gray hogback of San Gorgonio rises grandly across the deep trough of San Gorgonio Pass. Eastward sprawls the drab tawniness of the Colorado Desert and its debris-strewn hills. Southeast lies the shining platter of the Salton Sea and beyond, in the distant haze, is Mexico. But what gives the panorama a final touch of grandeur is the gigantic north rampart, plunging in sheer cliffs and castellated ridges to Coachella Valley, nearly two miles below. It is truly the altar of the Gods!

To the early Native Americans of Southern California, San Jacinto was a sacred mountain. The Cahuillas knew it as "Aya Kaich," meaning "smooth cliffs," the home of the meteor Dakush, legendary founder of the Cahuilla people. The Luisenos called it "Yamiwa," the Serranos "Sovovo." Even the far-away Gabrielinos revered it as "Jamiwu." The Spanish padres supposedly gave it the name "San Jacinto," after an outlying stock ranch of Mission San Luis Rey, which in turn was named for the fifteenth-century martyr Saint Hyacinth of Silesia. Lieutenant Robert S. Williamson's Pacific Railroad survey party passed under its towering face in 1853, mistakenly calling it "San Gorgonio" and misjudging its heights as 6000–7000'. Two years later, Dr. Thomas Antisell of Lieutenant John G. Parke's railroad survey party corrected Williamson's error. Antisell's report of 1855 contains the first written reference to the peak as "San Jacinto."

Who made the first ascent of San Jacinto Peak will probably never be known. Most likely it was a Cahuilla hunter, centuries before the arrival of

---

1 The quote is good, but the author could find no evidence that Muir ever climbed San Jacinto Peak.

the Europeans. The earliest climb on record was made in 1874 by a person identified only as "F. of Riverside" (story in *San Diego Union* of Sep. 16, 1874), who rode a horse up most of the way and scrambled the last 1000' on foot. In 1878 the peak was climbed by Lieutenant George M. Wheeler's U.S. Army survey party, which used the summit for a triangulation station and calculated its height at 10,987' above sea level.

In 1897 Edmund T. Perkins of the United States Geological Survey lugged a 60-pound plane table and theodolite to the top without benefit of trail, and corrected the elevation to 10,805'. Perkins' work was amazingly accurate—today's official height, determined by instruments far superior to those he used, is 10,804'. The first trail to the summit was forged by the U.S. Coast and Geodetic Survey in 1898 in order to install a heliograph for signaling to parties on other Southern California peaks. This trail was the forerunner of the present Devils Slide–Round Valley–San Jacinto Peak route. Since then, thousands have made the ascent via this trail and other footpaths constructed by the CCC during the mid-1930s. The stone shelter cabin just below the summit was built by the CCC in 1936.

This trip takes the most direct and the most traveled route from Idyllwild to the summit. It is an arduous 8-mile pull, but one of the most scenic and rewarding mountain paths in Southern California. You climb rock-ribbed slopes, cross chaparral thickets, pass through dense forest, and pause at bubbling springs. The higher you climb, the more glorious the vista. Halfway up, high on the mountainside, you pass a spot of lush grasses ribboned with trickling rills of icy water. This is Wellman Cienaga, named for Frank Wellman, a part Irish and part English character who herded cattle on the mountain in the 1890s. Beyond Wellman's you enter a world of weather-toughened lodgepole, sky-piercing granite crests, and thin cold air—the alpine rooftop of Southern California.

Description

From Highway 243 in Idyllwild just below the ranger station, turn northeast on North Circle Dr. Drive 0.7 mile, passing Nomad Ventures (a good outdoors and climbing shop). At the 4-way intersection, turn right on South Circle Dr. Proceed 0.1 mile, then turn left on Fern Valley Road. After 1.7 miles, reach a small parking area for the Ernie Maxwell Scenic Trail. Continue 0.1 mile up the hill to the outhouse and larger parking area of Humber Park (**GPS SB67**).

Climb the Devils Slide Trail, which starts at the top of the parking area, to Saddle Junction, 2.5 miles (see Hike 67 for details). At Saddle Junction, take the leftmost trail, leading north and marked by a sign indicating SAN JACINTO PEAK. You climb, through a forest of Jeffrey pine and white fir, up the bouldered ridge that forms the northeast wall of the Strawberry Valley amphitheater. Views into the valley and across to Lily Rock and Tahquitz

Peak are impressive. The trail then winds along the mountainside to a junction with the lateral trail to Strawberry Cienaga (see Hike 65), 2 miles from Saddle Junction.

Continue straight ahead (north), through lodgepole pine and white fir. The footpath rounds the head of Willow Creek to the grassy patch of Wellman Cienaga, 0.7 mile. Here is the last running water before the summit. Beyond Wellman's, you climb through thickets of manzanita and chinquapin to Wellman Divide, 0.5 mile, high on the ridge between Round and Tahquitz valleys. Here is a trail junction—left to the summit, right to Round Valley. If you're doing the climb in one day, go left. (If it's a two-day venture, your best overnight camp is in Round Valley—go right and descend to Round Valley Trail Camp, 1 mile.) Going the summit route (left), the trail climbs through a silent forest of lodgepole pine, then makes a long switchback up the southeast slope of San Jacinto Peak, through dense chinquapin and manzanita, to the ridgetop between Jean and San Jacinto peaks, 2 miles. Here you meet the abandoned trail coming up from the Tamarack and Round valleys. Go left, continuing up the mountain. You now make a long switchback up the southeast slope of San Jacinto Peak, through dense chinquapin and manzanita, to the ridgetop between Jean and San Jacinto peaks, 1 mile. Here you meet the San Jacinto Peak Trail. (The main trail continues down to Little Round Valley and Deer Springs—see Hike 66). Turn right and climb through an open lodgepole forest, past the stone shelter cabin, to the boulder-strewn summit, 0.2 mile.

Return the same way. Or take the roundabout route back through Round Valley and across Hidden Lake Divide (see Hike 70). With a 2-mile car shuttle, descend the Deer Springs Trail to Idyllwild (see Hike 66). Or take the aerial tramway down to Palm Springs with an across-the-range car shuttle (see Hike 85).

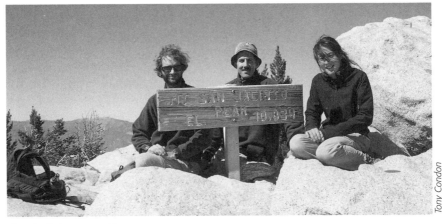

San Jacinto summit

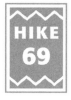

JEAN PEAK AND MARION MOUNTAIN

Hike Length: 16 miles round trip; 4600' elevation gain
Difficulty: Strenuous
Season: June–October
Topo map: *San Jacinto Peak* (7.5'),
                    San Jacinto Wilderness (Tom Harrison)
Permit: San Jacinto Wilderness Permit required

Features

Edmund Taylor Perkins had a special way of immortalizing the women in his life. He named mountains for them. When the tall, good-looking topographer came into the San Jacintos in 1897 to map the range for the U.S. Geological Survey, he met a young school teacher camped with friends near today's Pine Cove. She was Marion Kelly of White Cloud, Michigan, described as "a wonderful woman, blue eyes, and a gentle nature." She was employed by the Indian Bureau at the Morongo Valley Reservation. The story goes that Miss Kelly fell deeply in love with Perkins, but he kept putting her off by saying he was married to his work. But he did think enough of the young woman to place her name on a nearby mountain peak—Marion Mountain. Another young lady was in Perkins' mind too, one he had met previously while surveying in northern California. She was Jean Waters of Plumas County, California. He put her name on the neighboring mountain—Jean Peak. Marion was destined to be disappointed. Jean was more fortunate: she and Edmund Perkins were married in 1903.

No trails reach to the twin summits of white granite that eternalize the memory of these two young women. To reach them, you must scramble across jumbo boulders and, in the case of Marion, climb a short but rather precipitous summit block. This loop trip is only for those in top condition and experienced in cross-country travel.

Description

From Idyllwild Ranger Station drive west 1 mile on the Banning–Idyllwild Highway (State Highway 243). Park on the north side of the road just above the County Park Nature Center and past a sign pointing to Deer Springs Trailhead Parking (**GPS SB64**). Drive the other car to Humber Park: From Highway 243 in Idyllwild just below the ranger station, turn northeast on North Circle Dr. Drive 0.7 mile to a 4-way intersection, then turn right on South Circle Dr. Proceed 0.1 mile, then turn left on Fern Valley Road. After 1.7 miles, reach a small parking area for the Ernie Maxwell Scenic Trail. Continue 0.1 mile up the hill to the outhouse and larger parking area of Humber Park (**GPS SB67**).

Take the Devils Slide Trail to Saddle Junction, then the San Jacinto Peak Trail to the point where it reaches the ridge-top just south of San Jacinto Peak, 7.5 miles (see Hike 68 for details). Leave the trail here and scramble across boulders, south along the ridge, through an open lodgepole forest. You drop 100' to a saddle, then ascend 300' to the pile of white granite that marks the 10,670-foot summit of Jean Peak. After signing the Sierra Club summit register, continue down the ridge, south, then southwest, over an intermediate unnamed bump to the granite outcropping that is the summit of 10,362-foot Marion Mountain. The granite block is not difficult, but climb with care. After signing in here, continue down the ridge, curving west, through some brush, to the Deer Springs Trail. (*Note:* do not try to descend southeast to Wellman Cienaga or south to the Strawberry Cienaga Trail from Marion Mountain—you will become tangled in dense, thorny chaparral.) Follow the Deer Springs Trail 4 miles south to Idyllwild County Park Visitor Center.

Alternatives to avoid a car shuttle are two: climb back over Jean Peak to the San Jacinto Peak Trail and descend the way you came; or drop southwest down the ridge from Marion Mountain to the Deer Springs Trail, then take the Strawberry Cienaga lateral trail (see Hike 65) back to the San Jacinto Peak Trail below Wellman Cienaga. Both of these options add about 4 miles to the total hiking mileage.

HUMBER PARK–ROUND VALLEY LOOP

HIKE 70

Hike Length:	15 miles round trip; 3600' elevation gain
Difficulty:	Strenuous (1 day), Moderate (2 days)
Season:	June–October
Topo map:	*San Jacinto Peak* (7.5'),
	San Jacinto Wilderness (Tom Harrison)
Permit:	San Jacinto Wilderness Permit required

Features

Southeast from San Jacinto's lofty crown, nestled in high hanging valleys ringed by jagged spurs of white granite, is an enchanting wonderland of green. Here, suspended 8000' above the desert, pines and firs grow tall and sturdy, lush meadows are waist-high with fern and azalea, lupines spot hillsides in their late-summer bloom of purple and pale mauve, and little singing streams flow clear and cold. In the heart of this high sylvan wilderness is Round Valley, an oval meadow of verdant grass, threaded by an icy-cold brook, surrounded by a dense forest of lodgepole pine. Here is the most popular trail camp in the San Jacinto high country, frequented by dozens of backpackers almost every summer and early fall weekend.

This trip makes a broad loop through this inviting wilderness beneath the high peaks, with an overnight stop in Round Valley. The entire hike is on good trail and can be done in one long day, if you're in a monumental hurry. But it's a much more enjoyable trip if you take the full two days and savor this superb bit of sylvan grandeur high on the rugged shoulder of the San Jacintos.

Description

From Highway 243 in Idyllwild just below the ranger station, turn northeast on North Circle Dr. Drive 0.7 mile, passing Nomad Ventures (a good outdoors and climbing shop). At the 4-way intersection, turn right on South Circle Dr. Proceed 0.1 mile, then turn left on Fern Valley Road. After 1.7 miles, reach a small parking area for the Ernie Maxwell Scenic Trail. Continue 0.1 mile up the hill to the outhouse and larger parking area of Humber Park (**GPS SB67**).

Climb the Devils Slide Trail, which starts at the top of the parking area, to Saddle Junction, 2.5 miles (see Hike 67 for details). At Saddle Junction take the trail fork leading northeast, marked WILLOW CREEK and LONG VALLEY. The 1.5-mile walk to Willow Creek Trail Camp passes through a forest garden of ferns shaded by tall Jeffrey pines, passing a side trail leading south to Skunk Cabbage Meadow. Here, on a forested bench above the stream, is Willow Creek Trail Camp. Beyond, the trail starts climbing northeastward, and in

0.5 mile it reaches a junction with a new lateral trail down to Laws Camp
and Tahquitz Valley. Continue straight ahead and within minutes arrive at
the boundary of Mount San Jacinto State Wilderness, marked by a handsome
sign. (California State Park signs are usually done in a more artistic manner
than Forest Service signs.)

The trail continues to climb higher on the south slope of the rocky divide
overlooking Tahquitz Creek, with splendid vistas over the latter and beyond
to the desert and the Santa Rosa Mountains. About 2.5 miles from Willow
Creek, the trail makes several switchbacks and reaches Hidden Lake Divide.
Just beyond, leading east, is the presently closed lateral trail to Hidden Lake
and Desert View. The little lake, just above the escarpment, has suffered from
overuse and needs time to recuperate, so please do not visit it. Continue
north on the main trail. In 0.25 mile you reach a junction with the trail leading northeast to Long Valley and the upper tramway terminal, 1 mile. Go left
(northwest)—the sign indicates ROUND VALLEY 2 MILES. The trail contours
through lodgepole pines, along the north slope of the divide overlooking
Long Valley, passes a junction with the other end of the loop trail from Long
Valley and the tramway, and reaches the lush green meadow of Round Valley.
Here, on both sides of the valley, are many lodgepole-shaded camping spots.

For the return trip, take the trail that leads west, upstream; a sign indicates WELLMAN JUNCTION 1 MILE. You climb 1 mile through lodgepoles, verdant grasses, and lupine to a junction with the San Jacinto Peak Trail. Turn
left (southwest) and descend the trail through Wellman Cienaga to Saddle
Junction, 3.3 miles (see Hike 68 for details). Then take the Devils Slide Trail
down to Humber Park.

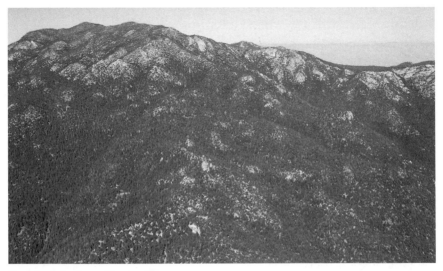

San Jacinto from the south

TAHQUITZ VALLEY

Hike Length: 7 miles round trip; 1700' elevation gain
Difficulty: Moderate
Season: June–October
Topo maps: *San Jacinto Peak, Palm Springs* (both 7.5'), *San Jacinto Wilderness* (Tom Harrison)
Permit: San Jacinto Wilderness Permit required

Features

Close under the granite spurs of Tahquitz Peak, nestled in a shallow bowl floored with forest and lush green meadow, is Tahquitz Valley. For the lover of pure sylvan beauty, this is the best the San Jacintos have to offer. Ferns and azaleas grow waist-high amid emerald grassland. Lemon lilies, crimson penstemon, purple lupine, and creamy buttercups add an enchanting dash of brilliance during early-summer bloom. Springs bubble up cool clear water and a musical creek threads the valley floor. Surrounding this mountain garden are dense stands of pine and fir.

Years ago, cowboys herded cattle up the notorious Devils Slide and into Tahquitz Valley to feed on the rich grasses. Frank Wellman is said to have built the first cabin here back in the 1890s. But the cattle have been gone for over 70 years and the old cabin has been removed, and nature's pristine beauty once again reigns in this lovely mountain basin.

This trip climbs the Devils Slide Trail and drops into this sylvan sanctuary. You can do it in one day, picnicking in the green, flower-bedecked turf, or make it a leisurely two-day jaunt, staying the night in one of the camping zones, indicated by yellow posts, in Tahquitz Valley.

Description

From Highway 243 in Idyllwild just below the ranger station, turn northeast on North Circle Dr. Drive 0.7 mile, passing Nomad Ventures (a good outdoors and climbing shop). At the 4-way intersection, turn right on South Circle Dr. Proceed 0.1 mile, then turn left on Fern Valley Road. After 1.7 miles, reach a small parking area for the Ernie Maxwell Scenic Trail. Continue 0.1 mile up the hill to the outhouse and larger parking area of Humber Park (**GPS SB67**).

Climb the Devils Slide Trail, which starts at the top of the parking area, to Saddle Junction, 2.5 miles (see Hike 67 for details). At Saddle Junction, take the trail leading right (southeast), marked by a sign indicating TAHQUITZ VALLEY. Proceed 0.75 mile through the forest of Jeffrey pine and white fir to Tahquitz Valley. Here is the Tahquitz Valley camping zone, with yellow posts indicating where you may camp. Water is always available here. Stop here or proceed 0.25 mile farther south, going right at a trail fork, to Little Tahquitz Valley and its camping zone. There's water here also. A left turn at the before-mentioned junction takes you to Reeds Meadow camping zone, with water from the stream. The water will need to be purified before drinking.

If you are making Tahquitz Valley your base camp and staying awhile, several interesting side trips are possible. You can climb by good trail to Tahquitz Peak Lookout (see Hike 73). You can descend Tahquitz Creek to Laws Camp and Caramba (see Hike 72), also on good trail. You can walk a short distance north to Skunk Cabbage Meadow (see Hike 67). Or you can scramble cross-country up Red Tahquitz for a breathtaking view of the Desert Divide country (see Hike 75).

Return the same way. An option is to take the trail to the roadhead above Saunders Meadow (see Hike 76).

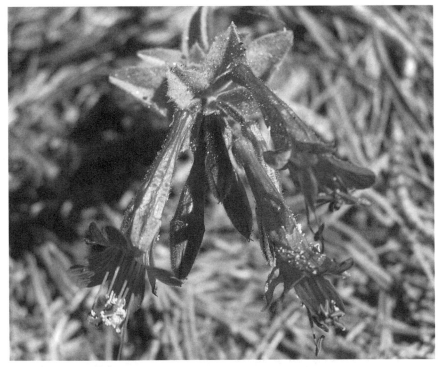

Penstemon (*Penstemon labrosus*)

CARAMBA

Hike Length: 13.5 miles round trip; 3300' elevation gain
Difficulty: Strenuous (1 day), Moderate (2 days)
Season: June–October
Topo maps: *San Jacinto Peak, Palm Springs* (both 7.5'),
San Jacinto Wilderness (Tom Harrison)
Permit: San Jacinto Wilderness Permit required

Features

Eastward from Tahquitz Valley, Tahquitz Creek descends in little tumbling cascades and swirling rapids for three meandering miles, then plunges abruptly off the eastern precipice to die in the thirsty sands of the desert. As the creek loses elevation, the character of the vegetation changes. Emerald grasses, ferns and flowering herbs gradually give way to willow thickets and clumps of bitter cherry and nettle. The adjacent forest cover changes too, from dense stands of white fir and Jeffrey pine to sparse Jeffreys and finally to hardy pinyon pine.

Winding through the Tahquitz Creek basin, from Tahquitz Valley through Laws Camp to the sudden dropoff just past Caramba, is a well-beaten trail, a pathway through some of the wildest high country in the range.

Laws Camp, near the junction of Willow and Tahquitz creeks, commemorates writer George Law, who built a cabin of shale rock with a ramada-type roof near here about 1916. Every summer for years, Law and his "little donkeys with their tinkering bells" would pack in to enjoy nature's solitude and find inspiration for his newspaper and magazine articles. The remains of his old cabin are almost gone, hidden on a rocky spur several hundred yards above Willow Creek.

Caramba is a little-used Spanish word meaning strange or unusual. The story goes that many years ago some cowboys camping here were terrified by weird sounds during the night and gave the place this unusual name.

This trip climbs over the Devils Slide and drops down Tahquitz Creek to the small trail camps at Laws and Caramba. Just past the latter, you are rewarded with a breathtaking vista over the desert. If you like your mountains primitive and unpeopled, this outing should suit your taste.

Description

From Highway 243 in Idyllwild just below the ranger station, turn northeast on North Circle Dr. Drive 0.7 mile, passing Nomad Ventures (a good outdoors and climbing shop). At the 4-way intersection, turn right on South Circle Dr. Proceed 0.1 mile, then turn left on Fern Valley Road. After 1.7 miles, reach a small parking area for the Ernie Maxwell Scenic Trail.

Continue 0.1 mile up the hill to the outhouse and larger parking area of Humber Park (**GPS SB67**).

Climb the Devils Slide Trail, which starts at the top of the parking area, to Saddle Junction, 2.5 miles (see Hike 67 for details). At Saddle Junction take the trail leading right (southeast), marked TAHQUITZ VALLEY and LAWS-CARAMBA. Proceed 0.75 mile through forests of pine and fir to Tahquitz Valley. In the valley take the trail forking left (northeast), marked LAWS and CARAMBA. The trail proceeds above the north bank of Tahquitz Creek, dropping 400' in 1.5 miles to Laws Camp, a small forested camping zone alongside Willow Creek. A lateral trail leads north from here to connect with the main Humber Park–Round Valley Trail (Hike 70), 1 mile. Beyond Laws, your trail follows the north slope high above Tahquitz Creek, then drops to Caramba, another small camping zone just above the eastern precipice—300' gain and 1000' loss in 2 miles from Laws. Just east of Caramba, you can scramble onto some large rock outcroppings for superb views over the desert face of the San Jacintos. But do not try to descend the precipice or Tahquitz Creek to the desert—many have become lost or injured trying. The Gordon Trail once went this way, but it has not been maintained for over 70 years, and is impossible to follow now.

Return the way you came.

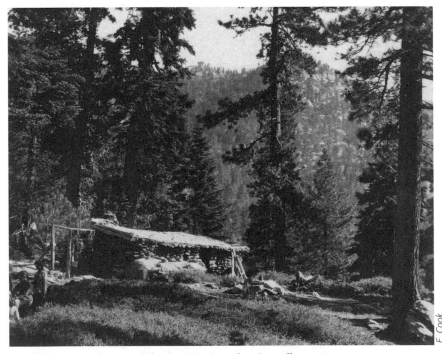

George Law's cabin, now long gone, in Tahquitz Valley—1921

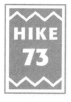

TAHQUITZ PEAK VIA SADDLE JUNCTION

HIKE 73

Hike Length: 8.5 miles round trip; 2400' elevation gain
Difficulty: Moderate
Season: June–October
Topo maps: *San Jacinto Peak* (7.5'),
San Jacinto Wilderness (Tom Harrison)
Permit: San Jacinto Wilderness Permit required

Features

Tahquitz Peak (8846') is the southern citadel of the San Jacinto high country. Its granite spurs and steep battlements rise impressively above Strawberry Valley on one side and Tahquitz Valley on the other. From the Forest Service lookout on its summit, you are rewarded with breathtaking panoramas over the southern half of the San Jacintos, with the Santa Rosas on the distant skyline.

Tahquitz Peak is named for the powerful evil demon of Cahuilla legend, who allegedly lived in a cave below the peak and came out at night to terrorize and devour Indians who ventured too close to his sacred mountain. The summit lookout tower, held up by steel beams, was built in 1938 to replace a more primitive wooden structure built around 1918. It is manned by volunteers during fire season, usually June–November.

Description

From Highway 243 in Idyllwild just below the ranger station, turn northeast on North Circle Dr. Drive 0.7 mile, passing Nomad Ventures (a good outdoors and climbing shop). At the 4-way intersection, turn right on South Circle Dr. Proceed 0.1 mile, then turn left on Fern Valley Road. After 1.7 miles, reach a small parking area for the Ernie Maxwell Scenic Trail. Continue 0.1 mile up the hill to the outhouse and larger parking area of Humber Park (**GPS SB67**).

Climb the Devils Slide Trail 2.5 miles to Saddle Junction (see Hike 67). At Saddle Junction take the far-right trail leading south, marked TAHQUITZ PEAK. In 1.25 miles through the forest, you reach Chinquapin Flat junction—covered, as the name implies, with a thick mantle of bush chinquapin. Go right again (southwest) and follow the trail up through chinquapin, lodgepole pine and a few limber pine to the summit lookout, 0.5 mile.

Return the same way, or take the South Ridge Trail down (Hike 77).

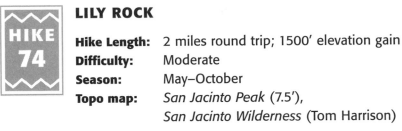

LILY ROCK

HIKE 74

Hike Length: 2 miles round trip; 1500′ elevation gain
Difficulty: Moderate
Season: May–October
Topo map: *San Jacinto Peak* (7.5′),
San Jacinto Wilderness (Tom Harrison)

Features

If you're starting up the Devils Slide Trail some summer weekend, chances are good that you'll hear faint shouts such as "On belay," "Climbing," "Off belay," and sometimes, "Falling." If you glance upward, you may be able to spot tiny, antlike figures clinging to vertical walls, now and then inching ahead with patience and care. These are rock-climbers testing their skill on the Yosemite-like dome of Lily Rock. Climbers prefer to call it by the more masculine-sounding name of Tahquitz Rock, but whatever you use, there is no doubt that this sheer-walled granite monolith offers the best technical climbing in Southern California. Almost every rock-climber in this part of the state has, at one time or other, improved his or her skill here.

The front walls of Lily Rock are no place for anyone not trained in climbing techniques. But for hikers who want to climb this striking natural feature, there is an easy route up the back side. This trip follows a very steep trail from Humber Park up and around to a saddle between Lily Rock and the serrated ridge leading to Tahquitz Peak; from here it is a short scramble to the summit. Wear boots with good tread.

Description

From Highway 243 in Idyllwild just below the ranger station, turn northeast on North Circle Dr. Drive 0.7 mile, passing Nomad Ventures (a good outdoors and climbing shop). At the 4-way intersection, turn right on South Circle Dr. Proceed 0.1 mile, then turn left on Fern Valley Road. After 1.7 miles, reach a small parking area for the Ernie Maxwell Scenic Trail (**GPS SB74**). If you reach the Humber Park parking lot and outhouse, you have gone 0.1 mile too far.

Take the prominent footpath marked ERNIE MAXWELL SCENIC TRAIL that leaves the southeast edge of the parking area and runs directly below Lily Rock. In 0.25 mile turn left on a narrow, unmarked trail that leads steeply up the slope towards the rock. The trail zigzags up the hillside, keeping just to the right of the prominent rockslide that extends down from the center of the rock. After 700′ of climbing, you reach what climbers call Lunch Rock, at the foot of many of the climbing routes. To your right (southeast) notice a worn pathway leading around the bottom of Lily Rock. Follow this trail— used by climbers descending from the rock—around the west face and steeply up the back side to the saddle between Lily Rock and the broken ridge leading up to Tahquitz Peak. From this saddle, scramble up easy granite ledges and slopes to the bald summit.

After taking in the fabulous view of Strawberry Valley and the high surrounding ridges, descend exactly the same way. Any other route is very dangerous.

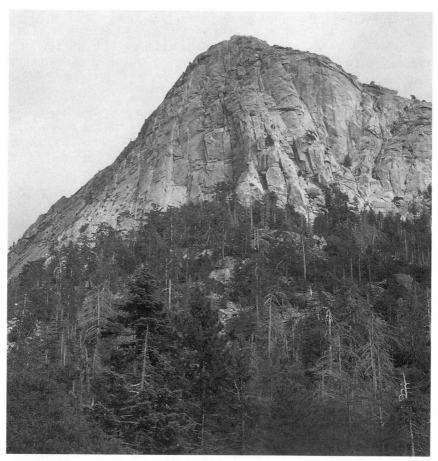

Lily Rock

DESERT DIVIDE

Hike Length: 16.6 miles one way; 2800' elevation gain
Difficulty: Strenuous (1 day). Moderate (2 days)
Season: May–October
Topo maps: *San Jacinto Peak, Idyllwild,*
                   Palm View Peak (all 7.5'),
                   San Jacinto Wilderness (Tom Harrison)
Permit: San Jacinto Wilderness Permit required

Features

South from Red Tahquitz Peak runs an extremely rugged mountain back-bone known as the Desert Divide, separating the high basin of Garner Valley from the desert-draining palm canyons to the east. The northern part of this backbone—from Red Tahquitz south to Antsell Rock—contains some of the wildest, most inaccessible mountain terrain in Southern California. Until the Pacific Crest Trail was carved through here in 1977, only the crude Sam Fink route penetrated this wall of granite spurs and saddles, brush-choked slopes and forested ledges.

The late Sam Fink, former Santa Ana fire captain whose avocation was mountaineering, was a living legend among Southern California hikers. One of his exploits was to build a trail along this foreboding mountain ridge. In 1967 Sam went up, by himself, with a saw and pruner and spent three days on the ridge, cutting brush and marking a route with red tags. This became known as "The Sam Fink Trail" and remained a hikers' route until the new stretch of the Pacific Crest Trail was cut and blasted through in 1977.

According to the Idyllwild district ranger, this stretch of Pacific Crest Trail over the Desert Divide was the most difficult route to survey and construct in all of Southern California. Parts of it had to literally be carved out of gran-ite walls by tedious drilling and blasting. The job required three years of strenuous effort.

The result is one of the best-engineered trails in California. A broad path-way and gentle switchbacks take the place of the steep, sometimes exposed, tedious scrambling of the old Sam Fink route. This trail trip takes the hiker over the northern, more spectacular section of the new footpath, from Tahquitz Valley to the Apache Peak–Spitler Peak saddle.

You can do it in one long, strenuous day, or, better, stay the night in Tahquitz or Little Tahquitz Valley and enjoy two days in this premier moun-tain wilderness country.

Description

The trip requires a car shuttle. Drive one car to the Humber Park parking area: From Highway 243 in Idyllwild just below the ranger station, turn northeast on North Circle Dr. Drive 0.7 mile, passing Nomad Ventures (a good outdoors and climbing shop). At the 4-way intersection, turn right on South Circle Dr. Proceed 0.1 mile, then turn left on Fern Valley Road. After 1.7 miles, reach a small parking area for the Ernie Maxwell Scenic Trail. Continue 0.1 mile up the hill to the outhouse and larger parking area of Humber Park (**GPS SB67**). Either park another car or arrange to be picked up at the Spitler Peak trailhead in Apple Canyon: Continue south on State Highway 243 to State Highway 74, then continue south 3.4 miles to Apple Canyon Road just before mile marker 074 RIV 62.75. Turn left and go 2.6 miles up the paved road to a turnout at the signed Spitler Peak (3E22) trailhead (**GPS SB78**). (*Note:* do not continue to the private ranches at road's end.)

From Humber Park, take the Devils Slide Trail to Saddle Junction (see Hike 67 for details). Here you reach a 5-way trail junction. Follow the Caramba Trail southeast (second from the right) to the edge of Tahquitz Valley to a second trail junction, then right (south) across Tahquitz Meadow and Creek to Little Tahquitz Valley, 1.25 miles from Saddle Junction. If you are making this a two-day trip, there are camping zones in both Tahquitz Meadow and Little Tahquitz valleys, with water that needs to be treated. To

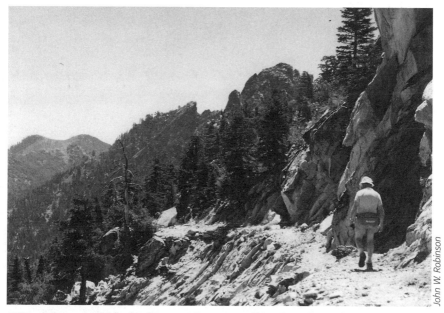

PCT on Desert Divide, looking south to Antsell Rock and Apache Peak

John W. Robinson

continue, proceed south up the Little Tahquitz Trail to its junction with the Pacific Crest Trail. Be certain to fill your canteens in Tahquitz or Little Tahquitz Creek; this is the last water until Apache Spring, 8.5 miles south.

Turn left (east) and follow the broad, well-graded PCT as it contours and climbs along the north slope of Red Tahquitz, through an open forest of lodgepole pine and white fir, then abruptly turns south around the east shoulder of the peak. Panoramic views open to the east, down over Andreas and Murray canyons to the deep trench of Palm Canyon and the desert beyond. Although much of the vegetation here was burned in the 1980 Palm Canyon Fire, it has grown back. Your trail gradually descends southward along the east slope of what is known as the Desert Divide, reaching a saddle between Red Tahquitz and South peaks, where you pass among the jagged granite crags with alternating views west to Garner Valley and Lake Hemet and east to the desert. The trail then climbs around the east flank of South Peak and drops in long, majestic switchbacks to the precipitous rock ridge north of Antsell Rock. The scenery here is more befitting the Sierra Nevada than Southern California. You pass well below the crags, traverse under the east face of Antsell Rock, and contour through a forest of bigcone Douglas-fir, white fir, and black oak to Apple Canyon Saddle. An old trail drops down Apple Canyon from here, but you don't take it; it has been closed because it traverses private property. Staying on the PCT, you climb the open slopes of Apache Peak, traverse around the east flanks a few hundred feet below the bare summit, and reach a junction with the Apache Spring Trail. The spring, which usually has water, is 1 mile down to your left (east). Continue south on the PCT down to the saddle between Apache and Spitler peaks. Here you can leave the PCT and turn west, descending the Spitler Peak Trail to Apple Canyon Road (see Hike 78 for full description), where your transportation should be waiting.

An option is to continue south on the PCT to Fobes Saddle, then right, down the Fobes Trail (4E02), to the Fobes Canyon Roadhead (see Hike 80). This option adds 1.25 miles to the trip.

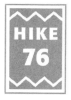

ERNIE MAXWELL SCENIC TRAIL

Hike Length: 2.5 miles one way; 300' elevation gain
Difficulty: Easy
Season: May–October
Topo maps: *Idyllwild, San Jacinto Peak* (both 7.5'),
San Jacinto Wilderness (Tom Harrison)

Features

This is an ideal family trip—level most of the way. The Ernie Maxwell Scenic Trail, named for the late Idyllwild conservationist and former editor of the *Town Crier,* contours along the mountainside above Strawberry Valley from Saunders Meadow to Humber Park. This easygoing footpath lives up to its name, winding through rich stands of pine, fir, and oak, with superb vistas over the densely wooded valley to the granite spurs of Marion Ridge. In spring wildflowers add a beautiful sprinkling of color. It is a fitting introduction to the Idyllwild country.

Description

From Highway 243 on the south edge of Idyllwild next to the Idyllwild School, drive up Saunders Meadow Road for 0.8 mile. Turn left on Pine Avenue, drive 0.2 mile, then turn right on Tahquitz View Drive for 0.5 mile, passing the South Fork Trail road junction, to the beginning of the ERNIE MAXWELL SCENIC TRAIL, so marked by a small sign to the right of the roads (**GPS SB76**). Parking is limited to a few wide spots along the road. You finish at Humber Park, so have someone meet you there or employ a car shuttle. To reach Humber Park, return to Highway 243 and turn northeast on North Circle Dr just below the ranger station. Drive 0.7 mile to a 4-way intersection, then turn right on South Circle Dr. Proceed 0.1 mile, then turn left on Fern Valley Road. After 1.7 miles, reach a small parking area for the Ernie Maxwell Scenic Trail (**GPS SB74**). If you reach the Humber Park parking lot outhouse, you have gone 0.1 mile too far.

Follow the well-built trail as it winds along the slope through beautiful forest. It is mostly level going, with gentle ups and downs here and there. The prominent feature ahead is Lily Rock, which looms more massively as you get nearer. The final 0.5 mile is gentle uphill, with 2 switchbacks just before reaching Humber Park.

You can do this trail the other way—from Humber Park to Tahquitz View Drive—even more easily.

TAHQUITZ PEAK VIA SOUTH RIDGE TRAIL

HIKE 77

Hike Length: 7 miles round trip; 2300' elevation gain
Difficulty: Moderate
Season: June–October
Topo maps: *Idyllwild, San Jacinto Peak* (both 7.5'),
San Jacinto Wilderness (Tom Harrison)
Permit: San Jacinto Wilderness Permit required

Features

This trail trip climbs the steep south ridge to Tahquitz Peak, zigzagging up through stands of Jeffrey pine, white fir, and live oak, with chinquapin thickets and lodgepole pine near the top. Various points along the trail offer far-reaching vistas south over the Desert Divide country, and northwest over Strawberry Valley to Marion Mountain and its rocky spurs. Years ago, the route followed an old, steep footpath up from Keen Camp; old timers would hardly recognize today's well-graded trail.

Description

From Highway 243 on the south edge of Idyllwild next to the Idyllwild School, drive up Saunders Meadow Road for 0.8 mile. Turn left on Pine Avenue, drive 0.2 mile, then turn right on Tahquitz View Drive for 0.3 mile. Just before the road becomes dirt, turn right on South Ridge Road (5S11). Proceed 0.9 mile, passing several minor side roads, to the signed South Ridge Trail (3E08) parking area (**GPS SB77**). Follow the trail as it climbs to the ridge crest, then zigzags up the divide through rich forest. In 1.25 miles you reach a flat area laced with jumbo boulders—halfway, a good rest stop. Beyond, you climb steeply through chinquapin thickets and scattered lodge-poles, between granite gendarmes, to the summit lookout, 3.6 miles from the start.

After taking in the fabulous panorama over the southern half of the San Jacintos, descend the way you came. An option, with car shuttle, is to descend the Tahquitz Peak Trail to Saddle Junction, then go down the Devils Slide Trail to Humber Park (see Hike 73).

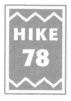

ANTSELL ROCK

Hike Length: 16 miles round trip; 2700' elevation gain
Difficulty: Strenuous
Season: All year
Topo maps: *Idyllwild, Palm View Peak* (both 7.5'),
San Jacinto Wilderness (Tom Harrison)
Permit: San Jacinto Wilderness Permit required

Features

Antsell Rock at 7679 feet is the crowning feature of the Desert Divide. Its imposing knob of multicolored rock can be seen from almost anywhere in Garner Valley. Antsell Rock is one of the very few peaks in the San Jacintos whose ascent involves more than a plodding walk up. Its nearly vertical upper ramparts give you a taste of the alpinist's exhilaration. It's what climbers call a "fun peak."

The peak was named by U.S.G.S. topographer Edmund Perkins in 1897–98. The story goes that Perkins ran across an artist painting mountain scenes at Keen Camp, an early-day resort just east of Mountain Center. The artist's name was Antsell and the mountain he was painting was this imposing rock knob, so Perkins labeled the knob "Antsell Rock" on his survey map.

The climb is not particularly difficult for those in good physical condition who have had experience on Class 3 rock. Boots with deep tread for traction on rock are strongly recommended. Take extra care on the descent, for that is when most accidents occur.

The old direct route up Apple Canyon to the Desert Divide, so long the nemesis of property owners in the upper canyon, is no longer open to hikers. You must now use the newly rerouted Spitler Peak Trail (3E22) from lower Apple Canyon.

The Desert Divide has made a remarkable recovery from the great Palm Canyon fire of 1980, which burned right up Andreas and Murray canyons to the crest. The chaparral has grown back as green as ever, and only a few blackened tree trunks remind you of the former devastation.

Description

Drive south on State Highway 74 3.4 miles from Mountain Center to Apple Canyon Road just before mile marker 074 RIV 62.75. Turn left and go 2.6 miles up the paved road to a turnout at the signed Spitler Peak (3E22) Trailhead (**GPS SB78**). (*Note:* do not continue to the private ranches at road's end.)

Follow the rerouted trail east, through oak and high chaparral, then northeast up the rock-ribbed slopes of Apple Canyon's east fork. You pass through open groves of Jeffrey and Coulter pine and the ubiquitous live oak as you climb steadily to the Apache Peak–Spitler Peak saddle on the Desert Divide and a junction with the Pacific Crest Trail, 5 miles.

Turn left (north) and follow the PCT up and around the east and north flanks of bare Apache Peak, passing a side trail that drops down the desert slope to Apache Spring, and then down 200 vertical feet to Apple Canyon saddle. (The old trail down Apple Canyon joins the PCT here.) Continue north on the PCT through a forest of black oak, white fir, and Jeffrey pine until it traverses the slope almost directly underneath and east of Antsell Rock. Here you must look carefully for a small duck and a climber's rough path leading steeply up the gully to your left. Leave the PCT and follow this route up unstable slopes to the top of the divide immediately southeast of Antsell Rock's summit block. The final 100 feet to the top is class 3 and not recommended for inexperienced hikers. To continue, scramble to the top of the large rock outcropping to your right, then step across and friction-climb the sloping granite to a steep, narrow gully. Follow the gully to the summit ridge, and on to the summit. Some may desire a rope belay on these final pitches. Return the same way.

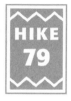

APACHE PEAK

HIKE 79

Hike Length:	12 miles round trip; 2600' elevation gain
Difficulty:	Moderate
Season:	All year
Topo maps:	*Idyllwild, Palm View Peak* (both 7.5'), *San Jacinto Wilderness* (Tom Harrison)
Permit:	San Jacinto Wilderness Permit required

Features

This trip climbs Apache Peak (7567') for a superb vista over the southern end of the San Jacintos and the desert canyons, then drops over the desert side to secluded Apache Spring. You follow the rerouted Spitler Peak Trail to the Desert Divide, then ascend the Pacific Crest Trail to the southeast slope of Apache Peak. Steep but clearly discernible lateral trails take you first up to the summit of Apache Peak and then down to Apache Spring.

Description

Drive south on State Highway 74 3.4 miles from Mountain Center to Apple Canyon Road just before mile marker 074 RIV 62.75. Turn left and go 2.6 miles up the paved road to a turnout at the signed Spitler Peak Trailhead (**GPS SB78**). (*Note:* do not continue to the private ranches at road's end.)

Take the Spitler Peak Trail (3E22) from lower Apple Canyon up to the Desert Divide and a junction with the Pacific Crest Trail (see Hike 78 for details). Turn left (north) and follow the PCT up to an unmarked but clearly discernible trail junction, 0.75 mile. Here you leave the PCT and scramble up a steep, rocky path to the bare summit of Apache Peak and its far-reaching vistas, 0.25 mile. Return the same way to the PCT, then take the lateral trail leading east and then northeast 500 vertical feet down the desert slope to Apache Spring. The little wooded spring always flows cold and clear, although in dry months it dwindles to a trickle.

Return the same way.

PALM VIEW PEAK

HIKE 80

Hike Length: 7 miles round trip; 2200' elevation gain
Difficulty: Moderate
Season: All year
Topo map: *Palm View Peak* (7.5')

Features

South from Apache Peak the Desert Divide gradually descends and loses its rugged character. Following along the crest of the long backbone from Apache south 13 miles to the head of Bull Canyon is the Desert Divide Trail, a hiker's avenue through waist-high chaparral and occasional clusters of fir and oak, with far-reaching views in all directions.

The Desert Divide country, particularly the southern half, is not well known to hikers. But it offers great opportunities for hiking trips, particularly in the fall-winter-spring season when the high country to the north is closed by snow. Sample it sometime; you won't be disappointed.

This trip accesses the Desert Divide Trail (PCT) from Fobes Canyon, formerly blocked to public access by a locked gate and the private property of Fobes Ranch. The trail (4E02) lies just east of the ranch boundary and offers easy access to Fobes Saddle, a low gap on the long Desert Divide. From the saddle, you climb southeast on the view-rich PCT to Palm View Peak. The panoramas are magnificent in all directions—the tawny Coachella Valley to the east, Garner and Anza valleys to the west, and on the northern skyline the San Jacinto high country, covered by its snowy mantle through spring.

Description

From State Highway 74, 6.8 miles southeast of Mountain Center and just past mile marker 074 RIV 66.00, turn left (northeast) onto the fair dirt Fobes Ranch Road (6S05). Stay left at a fork in 0.4 mile, then follow it across the Garner Valley for 3.2 miles to another junction. The main road goes north to Fobes Ranch (private); you turn right and proceed 0.4 mile to the signed Fobes Trailhead (**GPS SB80**). Parking is limited to three or four vehicles; you may have to park a short distance below the trailhead.

Proceed up the gently graded Fobes Trail (4E02), through waist-high chaparral and, higher up, through a small open grove of Jeffrey pines to a junction with the PCT at Fobes Saddle, 1.5 miles. Turn right (southeast) and follow the PCT as it climbs to a grassy bench, 2 miles from the low saddle. Halfway across the grassy area, veer left, off trail, through a grove of black oak and white fir, to the hidden summit of Palm View Peak (7162'). (The peak is misnamed—there are no palms nearby and the view from the wooded top is nonexistent.)

Return the same way. Or, you have several options. If your desire is to bag more peaks, you can follow the PCT north from Fobes Saddle and scramble to the summit of Spitler Peak (7440'), and/or Apache Peak (7567'), adding 4 and 6 miles respectively to the round trip. With a car shuttle, you can descend via the Spitler Peak Trail to Apple Canyon (see Hike 79) or the Morris Trail to Morris Ranch Road. Any way you do it, you're bound to enjoy this sample of the scenic Desert Divide country.

CEDAR SPRING

HIKE
81

Hike Length: 5.5 miles round trip; 1700' elevation gain
Difficulty: Moderate
Season: All year
Topo maps: *Palm View Peak, Butterfly Peak* (both 7.5')

Features

On both sides of the Desert Divide are a number of little springs trickling cold water. Cedar Spring, on the desert slope of the ridge, shaded by masterful incense-cedars and black oaks, is one of the nicest of these water sources. Just below the spring, in a shaded recess, is a small campsite much favored by hunters and Boy Scout groups.

This short trail trip climbs over the Desert Divide from Morris Ranch Road and drops into this little sylvan sanctuary with its ribbon of running water. It's best as a spring trip, when the water flows abundantly and the hillside is damp from spring rains.

Description

From State Highway 74, 8.6 miles south of Mountain Center in the Garner Valley and just beyond mile marker 074 RIV 67.75, turn left (northeast) onto the paved Morris Ranch Road (6S53). Follow it up 3.7 miles, passing the Joe Sherman Girl Scout Camp, to the signed Cedar Springs Trailhead (4E17) on the right (**GPS SB81**). (If you reach Morris Ranch, you've driven 0.25 mile too far.)

Proceed on foot up the trail to an oak-dotted valley, 0.5 mile. At the head of the miniature valley, pick up a trail that switchbacks up the chaparral-coated slope to a saddle on the Desert Divide, 1 mile. Here is a 4-way junction. Go northeast on a trail marked CEDAR SPRING and drop down the desert-facing slope 0.75 mile through chaparral, contouring north after 0.5 mile, to Cedar Spring, located in a forested crease in the mountainside. There is an unimproved campsite 100' below the spring, on a small shaded bench.

Return the same way. Or, from the 4-way trail junction, follow the PCT north to Palm View Peak and on to the Fobes Canyon roadhead (see Hike 80), adding 3 miles to the trip and requiring a car shuttle.

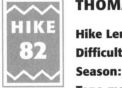

THOMAS MOUNTAIN

Hike Length: 12 miles round trip; 2100' elevation gain
Difficulty: Moderate
Season: All year
Topo map: *Anza* (7.5')

Features

The Ramona Trail climbs from Garner Valley over Thomas Mountain and down to the Ramona Indian Reservation, named, of course, after the beautiful Native American girl in Helen Hunt Jackson's famous novel. This trip takes the Ramona Trail to the crest of the divide, then follows the Thomas Mountain fire road northwest to the summit. En route you climb slopes dense with chaparral (mainly red shank) and reach into Jeffrey pine forest that covers the crown of the mountain, passing little Tool Box Spring and its primitive trail camp. There is water here usually the year round.

Description

From State Highway 74, in Garner Valley 8.1 miles south of Mountain Center just beyond mile marker 074 RIV 67.25, turn right into the Ramona Trail parking area (**GPS SB82**).

Follow the well-marked trail (3E26) as it switchbacks and climbs up the chaparral-coated mountainside.

As you climb higher, fine views open up over the Garner Valley, with the San Jacintos and Desert Divide country beyond. After 1.5 miles, you begin encountering Jeffrey pines, a welcome change from the shadeless red shank, manzanita, and mountain mahogany. In 2 miles your trail enters the forest and, a short distance higher, reaches Tool Box Spring and its welcome water seeping from the tank and the protruding pipe. From the spring, continue up the trail to Tool Box Campground, 3.5 miles from the highway. When you reach the crest of Thomas Mountain's long hogback, turn right onto Forest Road 6S13 and follow it northwest to primitive Thomas Mountain Campground and the summit, 6 miles from the start. The Forest Service has removed the fire lookout tower that long stood on the summit.

Return the same way. Or someone could drive up Thomas Mountain Road (reached from State Highway 74, 1 mile south of Lake Hemet turn-off) to meet you on top. Another option is to descend the other half of the Ramona Trail southwest to the Indian Reservation. Obtain permission before doing this.

CAHUILLA MOUNTAIN

Hike Length: 5 miles round trip; 800' elevation gain
Difficulty: Moderate
Season: November–June
Topo map: *Cahuilla Mountain* (7.5')

Features

Cahuilla Mountain, its stony battlements facing southward, rises in lonely isolation above Cahuilla Valley, 10 miles southwest of the San Jacintos proper. The mountain is seldom visited nowadays, yet it is the setting for the climax of one of the most famous novels of early-day California. The novel, of course, is Helen Hunt Jackson's *Ramona*, published in 1884.

High on the mountain, on a small flat between the summits of Cahuilla and Little Cahuilla, once lived Juan Diego, his wife Ramona Lubo, and their small child. Juan Diego, a Mountain Cahuilla who often did odd jobs for nearby white settlers, had fashioned a small cabin, a garden, and a few fruit trees alongside a spring here. He was known to those in the valley as friendly but "loco," whose occasional mental lapses caused him to do erratic things.

One day he returned home from sheep shearing in the San Jacinto Valley riding a strange horse. His wife, afraid he would be accused of stealing the horse, urged him to return it at once and get his own, which he had apparently left in the valley. Juan replied that he would as soon as he had rested, and fell asleep. He was awakened a short time later by the barking of dogs, and ran out to see what was causing the noise. A white man, Sam Temple, the owner of the horse that Juan had ridden home, rode up, and on seeing Juan poured out a volley of oaths, leveled his gun and shot him to death. After firing three more shots into the prostrate body, Temple took his horse and rode away. Ramona, who had witnessed the killing, ran with her baby on her back to the Cahuilla village and told what had happened. The next day the Cahuilla went up to the flat, brought Juan Diego's body to the village and buried it. Sam Temple was later tried for murder in the court of Judge Samuel V. Tripp and acquitted.

Here the story would have ended, soon forgotten, if Helen Hunt Jackson had not heard of it. Mrs. Jackson was concerned with the plight of Native Americans in the United States. In 1881 she had written *A Century of Dishonor,* a factual chronicle of white settlers' cruelty to Native Americans, but this book had not really stirred the public conscience. Now, in 1883, she was investigating Native American conditions in California for the federal government, and in the back of her mind was an idea for a novel to dramatize the sad situation. In the course of her work, Mrs. Jackson came to San

Jacinto and learned of the tragic killing of Juan Diego. Here at last was the long-looked-for episode around which could be crystallized the experiences and facts she had picked up in her studies. *Ramona* was conceived.

In the novel, the character Alessandro is patterned after Juan Diego. Jim Farrar is Sam Temple. (However, the beautiful Ramona of Mrs. Jackson's pen is in no way similar to Juan Diego's wife Ramona Lubo.) Although many of the episodes are pure fiction, the tragic climax where Farrar shoots down Alessandro with Ramona looking on is very close to what actually happened.

Ramona was an overnight success, and it achieved astounding popularity that has lasted to this day. The spotlight of public attention turned to the Cahuillas, and travelers came by the wagon-load into the Cahuilla Valley, some journeying up to lonely Juan Diego Flat, others seeking out Ramona Lubo. The plight of the Cahuillas, brought in sharp focus by *Ramona,* was lessened as the federal government stepped in to take a more active role in achieving justice for Native Americans.

Ramona Lubo died in 1922 and was buried beside her husband Juan Diego in the old Cahuilla cemetery that lies in the shadow of Cahuilla Mountain. Juan Diego Flat has been almost forgotten and sees few visitors nowadays. The access road, a small section of which crosses private property, is now open to the public.

This trip relives these stirring events of the past as it visits Juan Diego Flat and climbs to the top of Cahuilla Mountain for a breathtaking view over the country of Ramona and the Cahuillas.

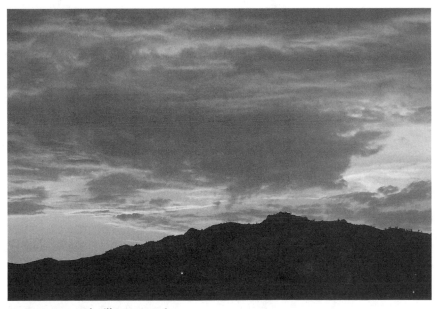

Sunset over Cahuilla Mountain

Description

West of the town of Anza on State Highway 371 near mile marker 371 RIV 68.0 at the sign for Cahuilla Mountain Trail (2E45), turn right (north) onto Cary Road. Cary Road eventually changes name to Tripp Flats Road. At a signed junction in 3.6 miles, turn left onto the dirt Forest Service Road 6S22. Drive up to Juan Diego Flat, 2.4 miles, to the beginning of the Cahuilla Mountain Trail (2E45), on your left, close to phone lines overhead (**GPS SB83**). A sign on your left indicates the trailhead. Park in the small clearing on your right.

Follow the distinct, well-graded trail up the northeast slope of the mountain, through an elfin forest of manzanita, to the ridgetop. The trail then crosses to the west side of the mountain, drops about 200 feet, contours, climbs through an open forest of black oak and Jeffrey pine, and arcs back to the 5635' summit, 2.5 miles. Or is it the true summit? The trail ends here and there is a summit register, but a point about 0.5 mile to the south appears to be as high, or perhaps a few feet higher. About 0.25 mile to the north there is another bump that looks equally high.

After taking in the superb vista east over the Anza Valley—the route taken by the great pathfinder Juan Bautista de Anza two centuries ago, and the long hogback of Palomar Mountain to the southwest—return the way you came.

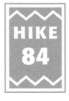

LONG, ROUND AND TAMARACK VALLEYS

HIKE 84

Hike Length:	5 miles round trip; 600' elevation gain
Difficulty:	Easy
Season:	May–October
Topo map:	*San Jacinto Peak* (7.5'),
	San Jacinto Wilderness (Tom Harrison)
Permit:	San Jacinto Wilderness Permit required

Features

From lower Chino Canyon, just above Palm Springs, the spectacular Palm Springs Aerial Tramway hauls visitors from palms to pines in a matter of a few short minutes. For hikers, this is the easy way to enter Mount San Jacinto State Park. From 8516-foot Mountain Station, the tramway's upper terminus, trails lead into the heart of the high wilderness.

This pleasant trip takes the wooded trail through upper Long Valley to the beautiful, though overused, green oasis of Round Valley. You can enjoy a picnic lunch along the crystal stream in Round Valley or under the tamarack (really lodgepole pines) in Tamarack Valley.

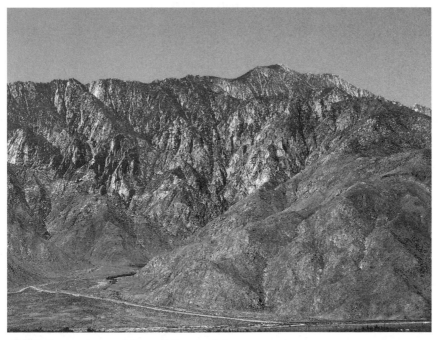

Chino Canyon on east face of San Jacinto

Description

From State Highway 111, 8.5 miles south of Interstate 10 at the northern edge of Palm Springs, turn west up Tramway Road and drive 2 miles to Valley Station, the lower terminus of the tramway (**GPS SB84**). The tramway operates daily, starting at 10 A.M. Monday–Friday; 8 A.M. Saturday, Sunday, and holidays. At the time this guide was written, last return is 9:45 P.M. Ride the tramway to Mountain Station, the upper terminus just above Long Valley. Round-trip tickets are $21.50. Visit www.pstramway.com or call 888-515-TRAM for more information.

From Mountain Station, proceed down the cement walkway into the Long Valley picnic area, then take the trail leading west, next to the ranger station, marked ROUND VALLEY 2 MILES. Follow the well-graded footpath as it leads up Long Valley Creek, through a rich forest of sugar pine and white fir. After a mile the trail veers left (southwest) and climbs into a lodgepole forest. In another 0.75 mile, you reach the Hidden Lake Divide–Willow Creek–Saddle Junction Trail (see Hike 70); continue west 0.25 mile to Round Valley. Here is a well-used campground and a 3-way trail junction. Turn right (north); the sign indicates TAMARACK VALLEY. You pass the trail camp and wind through a lodgepole forest to the grassy clearing of Tamarack Valley and its small trail camp, 0.5 mile. Across the valley, dominating the skyline, is the needlelike summit of Cornell Peak (named for Cornell University of Ithaca, New York, alma mater of Robert T. Hill, geologist for the USGS mapping party of 1897–98). Don't climb it unless you're an experienced mountaineer. Return the way you came.

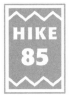

SAN JACINTO PEAK FROM THE TRAMWAY

Hike Length: 11.5 miles round trip; 2500' elevation gain
Difficulty: Moderate
Season: June–October
Topo map: *San Jacinto Peak* (7.5'),
San Jacinto Wilderness (Tom Harrison)
Permit: San Jacinto Wilderness Permit required

Features

The Palm Springs Aerial Tramway gives the hiker an 8000' head start on this desert-side route to San Jacinto Peak, leaving just 2300' to gain on foot. And this route climbs through some of the most verdant and inviting high country in the range—all on good, well-marked trail. You visit lush Round Valley, then ascend granite slopes dotted with lodgepole pines to the summit with the best view in southern California.

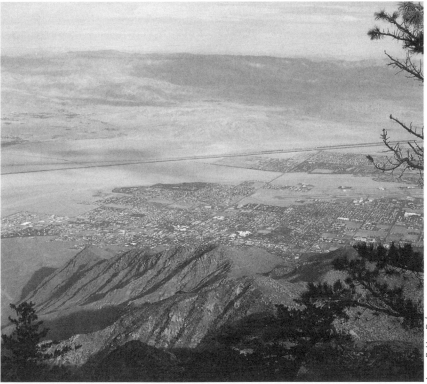

Larry B. Van Dyke

View of Palm Springs from the Aerial Tramway observation deck

Description

From State Highway 111, 8.5 miles south of Interstate 10 at the northern edge of Palm Springs, turn west up Tramway Road and drive 2 miles to Valley Station, the lower terminus of the tramway (**GPS SB84**). The tramway operates daily, starting at 10 A.M. Monday–Friday; 8 A.M. Saturday, Sunday, and holidays. At the time this guide was written, last return is 9:45 P.M. Ride the tramway to Mountain Station, the upper terminus just above Long Valley. Round-trip tickets are $21.50. Visit www.pstramway.com or call 888-515-TRAM for more information.

From Mountain Station, proceed to Round Valley, 2 miles (see Hike 84 for details). From Round Valley, your last dependable water, ascend the trail west—the sign indicates SAN JACINTO PEAK. You climb steadily through an open lodgepole forest to a junction with the Saddle Junction–San Jacinto Peak Trail, 1 mile. Turn right (north) and follow the well-used trail through the silent lodgepoles, then up a long switchback through dense manzanita and chinquapin, to the south ridge of San Jacinto Peak. Here you intersect the summit trail. Go right (north) and climb past the stone shelter building to the top, 300 yards.

Return the same way.

Note: The old trail, which cut a good 2 miles off the round trip from Long Valley to San Jacinto Peak, went from Round Valley north through Tamarack Valley and then up to a junction with the Saddle Junction–San Jacinto Peak Trail at what was once known as Wellman Junction, a mile short of the peak. The section of the old trail from Round Valley to Tamarack Valley is now open, and camping is again permitted at the latter. However, the section from Tamarack Valley to Wellman Junction was closed to protect a sensitive deer fawning area. It is overgrown with chinquapin, and brush debris blocks both ends. Whether that section of historic trail will ever be officially reopened remains to be seen. (Check with San Jacinto State Park authorities.)

LYKKEN LOOP

Hike Length: 4 mile loop; 1000' elevation gain
Difficulty: Moderate
Season: October–May
Topo maps: *Palm Springs* (7.5')

Features

The Lykken Trail is named after Carl Lykken, Palm Springs' first post-master. This trip leaves the western boundary of Palm Springs and heads up the east flank of the San Jacinto Mountains. It features a 180 degree view from north to south. All of Palm Springs is laid out before you. To the north and across the Coachella Valley, you can see the Little San Bernardino Mountains and the south end of Joshua Tree National Park. To the east you can see Palm Springs and beyond past the airport. You can watch airplanes take off and fly beneath you! To the southeast you see Palm Springs and some of the other cities of the Coachella Valley; Cathedral City, Rancho Mirage, and Palm Desert. To the south you see the Indian Canyons and Palm Canyon almost to its beginnings.

An added benefit at the end of the trip is that you can walk a few blocks to Palm Canyon Drive and have a bite to eat and something to drink at one of the very nice outdoor restaurants.

Description

Take Interstate 10 east over San Gorgonio Pass to Highway 111. Follow the highway south toward Palm Springs for 11.1 miles to Tahquitz Canyon Way. Make a right, go 0.1 mile, then turn right on Museum Drive.

The easiest way to do this trip is to start early in the morning and park on the street across from the Palm Springs Art Museum (**GPS SB86**). You can also pay $5 for all day parking in the lot adjacent to the Desert Fashion Plaza (across the street from the museum).

Walk south to Tahquitz Canyon Way and then jog left to Cahuilla Road and continue south to its end at Ramon Road (0.5 mile). There is also lim-ited public parking along Cahuilla Road. Turn right (west) and hike along Ramon Road for 0.4 mile to its end and the trailhead. There is no parking here but there is limited public parking on Camino Calidad for those who want to hike up the Lykken Trail and then return the same way.

Fifty yards up the trail from the trailhead, you will come to a fork in the trail. Take the least traveled path to the left that immediately leads to a series of steep switchbacks. From here to the end, the trail is well traveled and marked with white dots periodically painted on the rocks. The dots are par-ticularly helpful when hiking by headlamp for a sunrise or full moon trip.

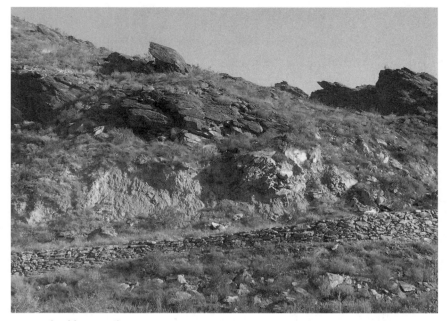

Start of Lykken Trail

Lizards scurry to and fro and you may startle a jack rabbit. Follow the trail up the ridges and then along the east flank of the San Jacinto Mountains enjoying the spectacular views. The trail passes through a field of barrel cactus. At a large cairn in about 2 miles, turn right and drop to the picnic area. Stop and enjoy the views and have a snack if you brought it. Unfortunately, vandals have been destroying the picnic tables.

From the picnic tables, head east and switchback down the steep trail to the museum. At one point, the trail goes uphill for 50 yards to bypass a rocky drop. Near the bottom, cross a paved driveway and come out at the signed trailhead at the northwest corner of the museum administration building by a small cactus garden.

Another trail climbs from the cairn upward to Long Valley at the top of the Aerial Tramway and to the peak of San Jacinto (see Hike 87). It is long, steep, hot, and dry. It is best not to venture upward from this point unless you depart before dawn.

SAN JACINTO VIA SKYLINE TRAIL

HIKE 87

Hike Length: 23 miles round trip; 10,700' elevation gain
Difficulty: Very Strenuous
Season: October–November
Topo maps: *San Jacinto Peak, Palm Springs* (7.5')
Permit: San Jacinto Wilderness Permit required

Features

After the San Gorgonio massif, San Jacinto is the second tallest peak around the Los Angeles Basin. This hike offers the greatest continuous elevation gain of any trail in the United States. It starts near sea level in Palm Springs and ends on the summit of San Jacinto. It is one of the testpieces for serious Southern California day hikers.

The Skyline Trail, also called the Cactus to Clouds Trail or Chino Trail, is not on most maps and is not officially maintained, but is in good condition and generally easy to follow unless covered in ice. The trail begins behind the in Palm Springs Art Museum and switchbacks up the ridge south of Chino Canyon to Long Valley near the Palm Springs Aerial Tramway. In Long Valley, it joins Hike 85 to the summit of San Jacinto. Most hikers descend the tramway and take a taxi or car shuttle back to the trailhead.

The Skyline Trail from Palm Springs to the Aerial Tramway, gaining 8000', is especially popular. At least five Southern Californians have hiked it nearly 200 times each! Cy Kaicener, 67 years of age, from Rialto, CA, has done the hike 193 times as of the time of this writing, and continues to hike it in the summer at 2 A.M. to beat the heat. He maintains a web site, www.hiking4health.com, with more information about the trail.

The Skyline Trail was originally a Native American footpath. It was improved by the CCC in the 1930s. The middle portion became overgrown with brush, but has recently been restored to good condition and now sees a good deal of foot traffic.

The trip is best done in late fall. Even in October, daytime temperatures in Palm Springs can exceed 100 degrees. Most of the trail is exposed to the sun. Start before dawn and carry at least five quarts of water. Wear plenty of sunscreen and a suitable hat. Carry salty food to restore your electrolytes. Strong and highly experienced hikers have suffered heat exhaustion and worse on this trail. Watch for rattlesnakes and don't get snagged by cactus. In winter and spring, the upper gully is notoriously icy and requires an ice axe and crampons.

Three other routes on the desert faces of San Jacinto are of historical interest: Tahquitz Creek, the Gordon Trail, and Snow Creek.

The Tahquitz Creek route climbs from Palm Springs up the extremely rugged gorge of Tahquitz Creek 6000' to Caramba Camp. It requires difficult climbing around waterfalls and nasty bushwhacking. The lower canyon is on the Agua Caliente Indian Reservation and may be closed to public access.

The Gordon Trail is another ancient Cahuilla footpath, improved by Dr. M.S. Gordon of Palm Springs in 1915–16 and the CCC in the 1930s. It has not been touched since and has completely disappeared beneath dense brush. It climbed from the mouth of Andreas Canon northwest up and over the ridge to Caramba Camp.

Snow Creek ascends the great North Face of San Jacinto. It starts in the town of Snow Creek and ascends the creek canyon directly to the summit of San Jacinto. The view of the route in winter and spring from San Gorgonio Pass on Highway 10 is awesome. The route involves Class 4 climbing around waterfalls and a huge chockstone in the canyon. The canyon is ravaged by avalanches after each snowstorm and accumulates a deep pack of snow. When the snow in the upper canyon is well consolidated, typically in April, the last six thousand feet are the longest snow couloir climb in Southern California. Unfortunately, the lower portion of the creek is on land owned by the Desert Water Agency, which has ceased issuing permits. Unless their policy changes, there is no legal access to this route.

Description

Take Interstate 10 east over San Gorgonio Pass to Highway 111. Follow the highway south toward Palm Springs. After 8.5 miles, you will pass

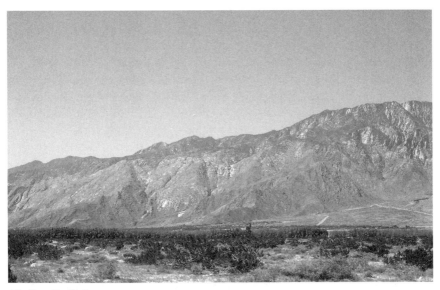

Skyline Trail view

Tramway Road on the right, leading 4 miles west to the Palm Springs Aerial Tramway, where you may wish to leave a car. Turn west up Tramway Road and drive 2 miles to Valley Station, the lower terminus of the tramway (**GPS SB84**). The tramway operates daily, starting at 10 A.M. Monday–Friday; 8 A.M. Saturday, Sunday, and holidays. At the time this guide was written, last return is 9:45 P.M. Ride the tramway to Mountain Station, the upper terminus just above Long Valley. Round-trip tickets are $21.50. Visit www.pstramway.com or call 888-515-TRAM for more information.

If you intend to drive to Palm Springs the previous night and get an early start, several inexpensive motels and a wide range of dining options are located on Palm Canyon Drive near the trailhead.

The Skyline Trail starts on the northwest side of the museum at a large sign at 480'. It switchbacks steeply up the hill and is clearly marked with white paint dots. After 1 mile, you will pass a 4-way trail junction; continue upward (west) for 11 more miles. Although it is not shown on maps, the trail is in good condition and is easy to follow. The Skyline trail picks up the top of the shallow ridge between Tahquitz and Tachevah canyons and follows this ridge through multiple desert ecosystems to a forested area and up a gully between a prominent rock outcropping on the left and a Coffman's Crag on the right before topping out in Long Valley at 8400'.

You have just climbed 8000 arduous feet. You can enjoy the shade, then walk over to the tram station and ride the tram down. If you have robust knees, you can retrace your steps back down the Skyline Trail. Or if time and energy permits, get a wilderness permit at the ranger station and top off water bottles. Then follow Hike 85 to the summit. After enjoying the view, return to Long Valley.

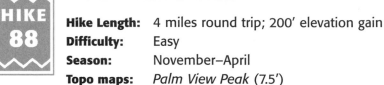

LOWER PALM CANYON

Hike Length: 4 miles round trip; 200' elevation gain
Difficulty: Easy
Season: November–April
Topo maps: *Palm View Peak* (7.5')

Features

The splendid palm canyons at the desert foot of the San Jacintos and Santa Rosas are a delight to behold. Thousands of California fan palms (*Washingtonia filifera*), their bright green fronds swaying in the breeze, crowd the canyon bottoms, seeking the life-giving water that tumbles down all-year streams. Rushes and other verdant water plants grow dense alongside limpid pools, completing the oasis effect that is all the more striking because the adjacent slopes are bone-dry and drab.

The daddy of all these green oasis canyons is Palm Canyon, running almost due south from Palm Springs to the Palms-to-Pines Highway. Somewhere around 3000 California fan palms grace the lower half of this canyon, extending from just below Hermits Bench almost to Palm Canyon Falls, a distance of 7 miles. Other groves of these palms extend short distances up many of the lower tributaries of Palm Canyon—Andreas Canyon, Murray Canyon, Fern Canyon, and the West and East forks of Palm Canyon.

For centuries before settlers arrived, the Cahuillas lived in these beautiful canyons. Relics of Native American habitation are still found along the banks and up the dry slopes—grinding holes, stone tools, faint traces of red pictographs. Today, most of lower Palm Canyon is the property of the Agua Caliente band of Mission Indians. Funds derived from the admission charges collected from visitors at the entrance gate go into the tribal treasury.

This trip follows a well-traveled trail that leads up Palm Canyon from the roadhead on Hermits Bench. It is a streamside walk through lush greenery, with arid canyon walls close on both sides. You have the option of extending the trip by wandering up some of the palm-filled tributary canyons. Do it in leisurely fashion to fully appreciate nature's unique contribution to the desert side of the mountains.

Description

From Interstate 10, take Highway 111 south into Palm Springs. The name changes to North Palm Canyon Drive. After passing through downtown, the road forks. Stay right as it becomes South Palm Canyon Drive. Continue to the toll gate at the entrance to the canyon, 15.2 miles from the Interstate (**GPS SB88**). At the time of this writing, the canyon is open from 8 A.M. to 5 P.M. From July 8–Oct 1, it is only open Friday–Sunday. The fee is $8, with discounts for students, seniors, and children. Call (800) 790-3398 for current information. After paying the entrance fee, proceed south 2.5 miles to the Trading Post at the end of the road on Hermits Bench.

Walk along the trail that drops into the canyon, then winds through the California fan palms, along the stream, up-canyon for about 2 miles. Beyond here, the trail follows the east slope before dropping back into the canyon farther up (see Hike 91). But you stop at the 2-mile point and saunter back down-canyon to Hermits Bench.

For a change of scenery on the way back, consider veering off to the right onto the Victor Trail at a signed junction 1 mile south of Hermits Bench. Follow the Victor Trail up the ridge along the east side of Palm Canyon for a beautiful overlook of the oasis. The trail drops down to join the Fern Canyon Trail. Turn left (west) and hike 0.1 mile back to Hermits Bench.

If you wish to explore these beautiful palm canyons further, trails lead up Fern Canyon, east from Hermits Bench, and up the East Fork, east from Palm Canyon 0.5 mile south of Hermits Bench. Or you can drive over to Andreas Canyon on your way out and explore the palm greenery there—the road leads west 0.5 mile from just south of the toll gate. Just remember you must be out of the canyons by 5 P.M., when the toll gate closes.

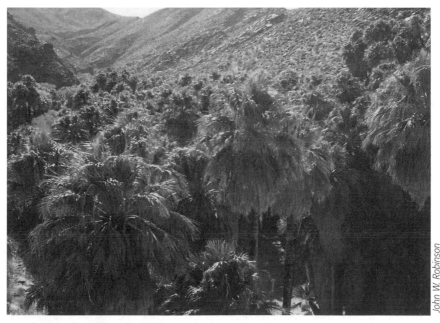

Washingtonia filifera, in Palm Canyon

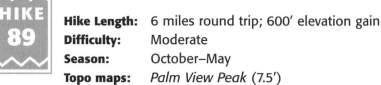

FERN CANYON LOOP

Hike Length: 6 miles round trip; 600' elevation gain
Difficulty: Moderate
Season: October–May
Topo maps: *Palm View Peak* (7.5')

Features

This is a hike into the hills east of Hermits Bench and into Fern Canyon. After crossing Palm Canyon Creek and walking up Fern Canyon for 0.25 mile, the desert traveler ascends a steep incline for 280 feet and is rewarded with beautiful views of Palm Canyon to the west and Palm Springs to the north and northwest. This is followed by a slight descent into Fern Canyon where it narrows and the south wall becomes vertical. Water seeps out along this shaded wall and supplies moisture to the hanging ferns growing on the wall. Once through this section, the traveler is back in the desert and continues east and south toward the Vandeventer Trail. When returning to Palm Canyon on this trail, one can enjoy views of the palm oasis from ridgeline 200 feet above the canyon floor. Hikers also have the option of taking shorter hikes up Fern Canyon Trail or Vandeventer Trail and then returning the same way.

Description

From Interstate 10, take Highway 111 south into Palm Springs. The name changes to North Palm Canyon Drive. After passing through downtown, the road forks. Stay right as it becomes South Palm Canyon Drive. Continue to the toll gate at the entrance to the canyon, 15.2 miles from the Interstate (**GPS SB88**). At the time of this writing, the canyon is open from 8 A.M. to 5 P.M. From July 8–Oct 1, it is only open Friday–Sunday. The fee is $8, with discounts for students, seniors, and children. Call (800) 790-3398 for current information. After paying the entrance fee, proceed south 2.5 miles to the Trading Post at the end of the road on Hermits Bench.

The Fern Canyon and Vandeventer Trails are well maintained and well marked. From the Trading Post at Hermits Bench, head east and down through the parking lot. Go to the gated, lower parking lot, around the hill, and to the left (at the north end of the lower lot). There you will see a poster board and marker post indicating the direction to the Fern Canyon, Victor, and Alexander Trails. Follow the trail to the stream crossing. On the other side, follow the well-defined trail up and into the lower part of Fern Canyon. In about a quarter mile, you will come to the junction of the Alexander and Victor Trails. The marker post indicates that the Fern Canyon Trail goes to the east into the hills. Ascend the steep incline, then drop back into Fern Canyon to view the hanging ferns in 1 mile.

Continuing up the canyon half a mile brings you to a marker post indicating the junction with the Wild Horse Trail. The Vandeventer Trail is to the east and south (as indicated by the marker post). While heading south, you will pass the well marked junctions with the Dunn Road Trail and the Hahn–Buena Vista Trail (which head to the east).

Once you reach the Vandeventer Trail, loop around back to the west and north to return to Hermits Bench.

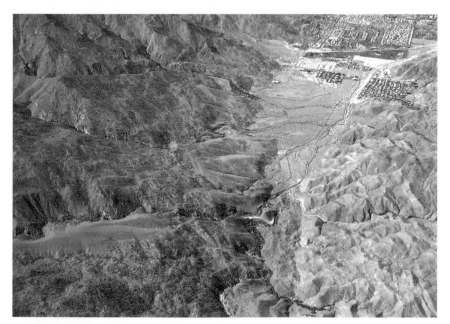

Hermit's Bench

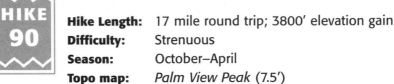

JO POND TRAIL

Hike Length: 17 mile round trip; 3800' elevation gain
Difficulty: Strenuous
Season: October–April
Topo map: *Palm View Peak* (7.5')

Features

The Jo Pond Trail is one of the highlights of the Coachella Valley. Starting in Palm Canyon, it ascends the Garnet Ridge to Cedar Springs, providing astounding views of the Coachella Valley, Salton Sea, and San Jacinto mountains, especially when the peaks are cloaked in their snowy winter mantle.

Despite what you might imagine, the Jo Pond Trail does not visit any standing bodies of water. Rather, it was named for a member of the Desert Riders, who was a strong proponent of trails in the Coachella Valley. The trail was completed in 1994.

A complication of this trip is that your vehicle must be out of the canyon by 5 P.M. when the gate closes. Watch the time carefully, or park outside the toll gate.

Description

From Interstate 10, take Highway 111 south into Palm Springs. The name changes to North Palm Canyon Drive. After passing through downtown, the road forks. Stay right as it becomes South Palm Canyon Drive. Continue to the toll gate at the entrance to the canyon, 15.2 miles from the Interstate (**GPS SB88**). At the time of this writing, the canyon is open from 8 A.M. to 5 P.M. From July 8–Oct 1, it is only open Friday–Sunday. The fee is $8, with discounts for students, seniors, and children. Call (800) 790-3398 for current information. After paying the entrance fee, proceed south 2.5 miles to the Trading Post at the end of the road on Hermits Bench.

Begin hiking on the aptly named West Fork Trail that ascends the west fork of Palm Canyon from Hermits Bench past waterfalls and flowering cacti. In about 2 miles, it reaches the Dos Palmas spring and picnic area, where the Pelton Trail heads northward. The West Fork Trail becomes the Jo Pond Trail and continues southwest for 3.5 miles to the Ponderosa Park picnic area. From here, the trail climbs Garnet Ridge for 4 miles to Cedar Spring. Portions of the ridge were burned in July 1994 and are regrowing. Your hike ends at a campsite in a stand of incense cedar at Cedar Spring.

From here, you can retrace your steps to Hermits Bench. Or, better yet, with a car shuttle, you can continue a mile to the crest of the Desert Divide where you cross the Pacific Crest Trail. Then switchback 2 more miles down the Cedar Springs Trail to the Morris Ranch trailhead in the Garner Valley (see Hike 81).

PALM CANYON TRAVERSE

HIKE 91

Hike Length:	18 miles one way; 3500' elevation loss
Difficulty:	Strenuous (1 day), Moderate (2 days)
Season:	November–April
Topo maps:	*Palm View Peak, Butterfly Peak,* and *Toro Peak* (all 7.5')

Features

This trip, best done as an overnight backpack, descends the length of Palm Canyon from Ribbonwood on the Palms-to-Pines Highway to Hermits Bench, 14 mostly downhill miles. Besides some spectacular canyon scenery, another highlight is the rich and varied desert flora. You start down through Upper Sonoran vegetation—slopes dense with red shank, mesquite, sage, yucca, and scattered junipers and pinyon pines. As you descend, Lower Sonoran flora becomes predominant—bisnaga, cholla, buckthorn, and hedgehog cacti, agave, ocotillo, goatnut, ephedra, and scores of other arid-zone plants. Then, alongside the creek, you meet the startling contrast of lush greenery—California fan palm, of course, supplemented by scattered cottonwoods, rushes, ferns, and grasses. It's a different world from the San Jacinto high country just a few miles above. Florally speaking, it's as if you had traveled from Canada to Mexico, the contrast is so pronounced.

A car shuttle is required for this one-way trip, made more complicated by the fact that you cannot leave your car at Hermits Bench or anywhere inside the toll gate (property of the Agua Caliente Band of Cahuilla Indians) overnight. Unless someone picks you up at the end, plan on hiking an extra 3.5 miles to the south edge of Palm Springs. But the rewards of this venture are so great that it is worth the extra complications.

Description

From the intersection of State Highways 111 and 74 in Palm Desert, drive up Highway 74 to Ribbonwood. Just past mile marker 074 RIV 77.85, turn north on Pine View Drive and proceed 0.2 mile to the end of the paved road (**GPS SB91**). Park here. Walk north along the dirt road through a ribbonwood grove. Pass a branch to the right, then make the next right at a blank steel trail marker, 150 yards from the car and just before the end of the main dirt road.

This is the beginning of the Palm Canyon Trail. Before heading down this trail, consider walking out to the clearing at the end of the main dirt road for a spectacular view of Palm Canyon. Twenty-five miles to the north you will see the dark green patches of trees and grass of Palm Springs

Arrange to be picked up at Hermits Bench, between 8 A.M. and 5 P.M. the following day. To reach Hermits Bench return on Highway 111 to Palm

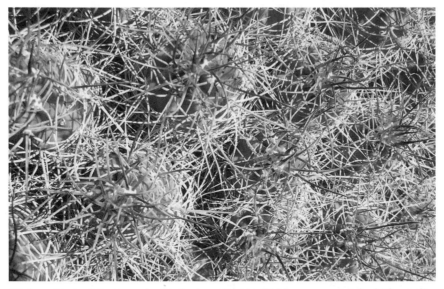

Mojave Mound Cactus, aka Hedgehog Cactus (*Echinocereus triglochidinatus*)

Springs. When the road turns right (north), stay left on South Palm Canyon Drive. Continue to the toll gate at the entrance to the canyon, 15.2 miles from the Interstate (**GPS SB88**). At the time of this writing, the canyon is open from 8 A.M. to 5 P.M. From July 8–Oct 1, it is only open Friday-Sunday. The fee is $8, with discounts for students, seniors, and children. Call (800) 790-3398 for current information. After paying the entrance fee, proceed south 2.5 miles to the Trading Post at the end of the road on Hermits Bench. Alternatively, you can leave another car at the south edge of Palm Springs, outside tribal lands, on South Palm Canyon Drive, and walk an extra 3.5 miles at the end.

The trail—in reality, jeep tracks—begins just before the end of the dirt section of Pine View Drive, to your right. This portion of the trail is not maintained but it is a wide cut through the ribbonwood and manzanita. About 0.8 mile beyond is a second junction. It is marked by a weathered wooden post with a wooden sign on it. The sign is lettered PALM CANYON TRAIL, 4E01, CANYON BOTTOM (arrow to the left), CANYON RIDGE (arrow to the right). At this junction you have the choice of staying on the ridge or descending into the canyon; both trails rejoin a mile down. After 1.5 miles, the jeep tracks become a trail. A half mile farther, you drop into the canyon bottom and walk close to the trickling stream. For the next 3 miles you mostly follow the canyon bottom, with detours here and there to get around rocky obstructions. You pass the entrances of Live Oak and Oak canyons, coming down from the Desert Divide country. Three hundred yards up the latter, out of sight around a bend, is Hidden Falls. A short, trailless side trip gets you to the foot of the falls.

About 5.5 miles from the start you pass a junction with the Live Oak Trail coming down from the Desert Divide (see Hike 92). Continue north down canyon; after 2.5 miles farther is Agua Bonita Spring, shaded by cottonwoods, a good overnight campsite. A short distance below here you enter tribal lands (overnight camping prohibited). Below Agua Bonita, the trail climbs southeast out of the canyon to get around the rocky gorge of Palm Canyon Falls. (There is no trail through this most spectacular section of Palm Canyon; hikers have reached the falls by scrambling up-canyon from below.) For the next 6 miles you follow the cactus-rich slopes above the east wall of the canyon, crossing several small tributary canyons. As you near Hermits Bench, you look down on splendid groves of *Washington filifera* palms, both in the main canyon and in tributary canyons to the west. The lush greenery amid the drab desert offers a scene of striking contrast. Finally you climb to Hermits Bench, where you either pick up your ride or walk 3.5 miles farther to Palm Springs.

DESERT DIVIDE AND PALM CANYON

HIKE 92

Hike Length:	17 miles one way; 2900' elevation gain
Difficulty:	Strenuous (1 day), Moderate (2 days)
Season:	November–May
Topo maps:	*Butterfly Peak, Palm View Peak, Toro Peak* (all 7.5')

Features

This backpack trip traverses the semi-arid southern end of the San Jacintos, climbing from Garner Valley over the Desert Divide, then dropping into upper Palm Canyon and ascending the latter to Ribbonwood. You pass through some rich chaparral country, and enjoy far-reaching vistas of snow-capped high mountains and tawny desert foothills. It makes an ideal winter or early spring outing.

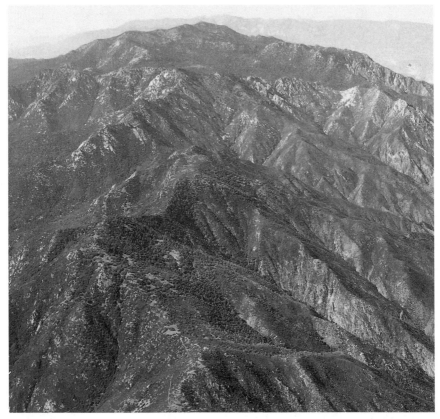

Desert Divide

Description

From State Highway 74, 8.6 miles south of Mountain Center in the Garner Valley and just beyond mile marker 074 RIV 67.75, turn left (northeast) onto the paved Morris Ranch Road (6S53). Follow it up 3.7 miles, passing the Joe Sherman Girl Scout Camp, to the signed Cedar Springs Trailhead (4E17) on the right (**GPS SB81**). (If you reach Morris Ranch, you've driven 0.25 mile too far.).

You will come out at Ribbonwood (see Hike 91), 10 miles farther down State Highway 74, so either shuttle a second car there or arrange to be picked up there upon completing your trip.

Hike east on the Cedar Springs Trail 0.5 mile to where it narrows, then pick up the trail that switchbacks up the chaparral-covered slope to a saddle on the Desert Divide, 1 mile farther. Here is a 4-way junction (see Hikes 80, 81). Go right (southeast) and follow the Pacific Crest Trail past Pyramid and Lion peaks, mostly through chaparral, with scattered groves of pine and oak, to a 4-way trail junction, 4 miles. You leave the Pacific Crest Trail here and turn sharp left (northeast), descending the Live Oak Trail to Live Oak Spring, 1 mile. There is usually water running out of a pipe here, and primitive camping facilities under the oaks. About 0.5 mile below Live Oak Spring the trail forks: the right branch is shorter and better maintained, reaching Palm Canyon in 2 miles. The left fork descends the ridge between Live Oak and Oak canyons, drops into the latter, and reaches the floor of Palm Canyon near Hidden Falls, 4 miles. Hidden Falls, spectacular in spring but usually dry by early summer, can be reached by a 0.5-mile scramble up Oak Canyon from Palm Canyon. Proceed up the Palm Canyon Trail (south) to Ribbonwood on State Highway 74, 5 miles via the shorter route, 7 miles via the longer. (See Hike 91 for Ribbonwood trailhead details.)

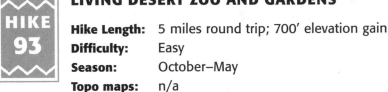

LIVING DESERT ZOO AND GARDENS

Hike Length:	5 miles round trip; 700' elevation gain
Difficulty:	Easy
Season:	October–May
Topo maps:	n/a

Features

After doing some of the more strenuous trips in the Palm Springs area, this trip is relaxing, educational, and fun in a different way. The Living Desert Zoo and Gardens is a beautiful desert environment set aside for a hike and an all-day learning experience for the whole family. In the Garden all plant varieties are labeled to help the visitor learn the name and its place in the desert environment. Plants are also grouped into living communities that represent desert regions around the world. For example, the Coachella Valley is a part of the Sonoran Desert and to the north is Mojave Desert. Animals roam freely in their own outdoor enclosures. Mountain lions, coyotes, golden and bald eagles, and desert big horn sheep are examples of the North American species displayed. Some of the African species on display are lions, jackals, hyenas, giraffe, and African antelope.

The Zoo and Gardens are open from 9 to 5 September 1–June 15 and 8 to 1:30 in the summer, though this hike is not recommended for the summer. You can do the hike and return to the Zoo and Gardens to take in the exhibits and read about the flora and fauna you just observed. Admission is $10.95, with discounts for children, seniors, and active military. Call (760) 346-5694 or visit www.livingdesert.org for more information.

Description

From Highway 111 in Palm Desert about 11 miles south of Palm Springs, turn south on Portola Ave. Go 1.5 miles and turn left at a sign into the main entrance (**GPS SB93**). The zoo has free parking. Alternatively, from Interstate 10, exit at Monterey Ave. east of Palm Springs, drive south 5.9 miles to Highway 111, and take it south 1.0 miles to Portola Ave.

This is actually three trips in one. The hiker can do the inner loop of 0.5 mile, the middle loop of 1.6 miles or the wilderness loop of 5 miles. All loops have signs posted describing various segments of life on a desert alluvial plain. The wilderness loop has the added bonus that you climb into a boulder-strewn canyon and then out and onto the flanks of Mt. Eisenhower, 700' above the floor of the Coachella Valley. From the flanks of Mt. Eisenhower all of the Coachella Valley is spread out before you. The San Andreas Fault and Joshua Tree National Park are to the north. There are beautiful views of Mt. San Gorgonio (elevation 11,502') to the northwest and Mt. San Jacinto (elevation 10,804') to the west. There is also a sheltered picnic table at this location to rest, snack, and soak in the views. A well maintained and traveled trail heading west takes the traveler along a ridge with more views of the above and the Zoo and Gardens. You then drop down onto the alluvial plain and back to the Zoo and Gardens.

At the entrance, be sure to ask for a map of the Wilderness Trail. From the entrance, walk past the gift shop and café and keep the model train exhibit on your right. Continue forward and slightly left through an open area (200 yards wide) to the Big Horn Sheep Hill. To the right of the Big Horn Sheep Hill will be other large enclosures for gazelles and the Arabian Oryx. To the left of the hill will be the trailhead. All loop trails are well marked with signs and on the handout map.

PART 3

The Santa Rosa Mountains

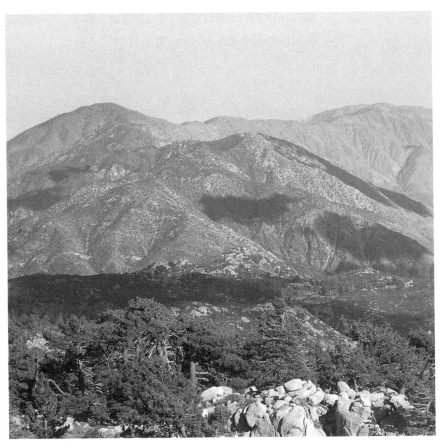

The Santa Rosas

Natural History of the Santa Rosa Mountains

Lay of the Land

South from the Palms-to-Pines Highway, the Santa Rosas rise as a sky island out of the desert foothills. Reaching elevations in excess of 8000' at Toro Peak and Santa Rosa Mountain, the high mountain backbone supports a rich forest of Jeffrey and ponderosa pine, white fir, and incense-cedar. A multitude of springs seep cold water down the slopes to the thirsty regions below. In summer, when the surrounding desert country swelters under the burning sun, this green oasis in the sky is cool and refreshing.

Plant Life

There are really two Santa Rosas. South and east from the lofty Santa Rosa Mountain–Toro Peak backbone, the range is lower and shows the strong influence of the desert. Here on the slopes and benches above 4000 feet, pinyon pine and California juniper are supreme, covering endless miles of mountainous terrain. On the north flank of the range is an ocean of chaparral, primarily shaggy-barked, olive-green red shank (also called ribbonwood). In the desert foothills and canyons to the east, west and south, Lower Sonoran vegetation takes over—tall and spindly ocotillo, yucca, chamise, barrel and cholla cacti, and waxy-green creosote. In some of the canyons are small oases of *Washingtonia filifera*, floral monarchs of the California desert. Except for the high backbone of Santa Rosa Mountain and Toro Peak, the Santa Rosas are primarily a desert range.

Wildlife

The desert Santa Rosas are the home of the largest herd of bighorn sheep in California, estimated at more than 500 head. These noble masters of the arid crags live mainly in the eastern and southern parts of the range, rocky regions where humans seldom disturb their living habits. Crucial to their survival are the handful of all-year springs that trickle from some of the pinyon flats and desert canyons. The easiest way to see and photograph bighorn sheep is to hide near one of these water holes and await their

233

appearance. (I have seen many in this manner.) Other large mammals common in the Santa Rosas are mule deer and mountain lion. The latter are seldom seen, but their large, unmistakable tracks betray their existence.

Perhaps the greatest appeal of the Santa Rosas is their relative isolation and primitiveness. Except for the forest road climbing to Santa Rosa Mountain and Toro Peak and, at the other end of the range, jeep tracks leading into Rockhouse Canyon, the range is devoid of roads. Trails are few, and most of those that do exist are unmaintained, ancient relics of the Cahuilla. You can have most of these mountains almost to yourself. They make for superb winter outings.

Fortunately, Congress has seen fit to protect most of the Santa Rosas. The Archaeological Resources Protective Act of 1979 makes it illegal to disturb or remove any of the Native American artifacts in these culturally rich mountains. The 20,160-acre Santa Rosa Wilderness, created by the California Wilderness Act of 1984, protects most of the northern Santa Rosas that are within San Bernardino National Forest.

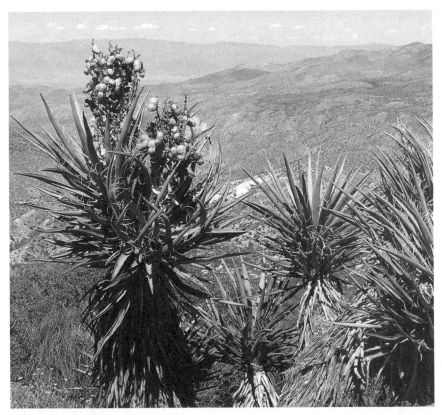

Fruity Yucca on Sawmill Trail

Thanks to the efforts of the Sierra Club and other activists, and with the strong support of Congresswoman Mary Bono (R) of Palm Springs and California Senator Diane Feinstein (D), the mammoth Santa Rosa and San Jacinto Mountains National Monument was established when President Bill Clinton signed the enabling act in October 2000. The 272,000-acre national monument encompasses most of the desert side of the Santa Rosas and San Jacintos and safeguards endangered bighorn sheep and desert tortoises. This is the first Congressional designated national monument under the supervision of the Bureau of Land Management.

A wilderness permit is presently not required to enter the Santa Rosa Wilderness or the Santa Rosa and San Jacinto Mountains National Monument, but may be so in the future if overuse threatens to degrade some of the canyons.

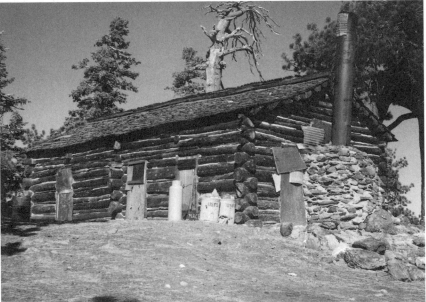

Desert Steve Ragsdale's cabin

Human History in the Santa Rosa Mountains

A Subsistence Life

Like the San Jacinto country to the north, the Santa Rosas were the ancestral home of numerous Cahuilla peoples. In Deep Canyon, on the northeastern slope of the range, were villages of the Western Cahuilla. Groups of Desert Cahuilla lived in spring-fed oases at the eastern foot of the mountains, above the shoreline of ancient Lake Cahuilla (today's Salton Sea). Mountain Cahuilla villages were numerous on the western slope of the range, particularly in Horse and Rockhouse canyons and on Vandeventer Flat. The Santa Rosas supplied these hardy people with the necessities of life—pinyon nuts, acorns, agave, yucca fibers, wild game, and water. Footpaths crisscrossed the range, traveling from spring to spring. Many of these ancient trails are still traceable today. In summer, whole villages would migrate into the mountains to gather food and escape the searing desert heat. About the only place in the Santa Rosas avoided by the Cahuilla was Toro Peak; there are stories that this highest mountain in the range was taboo, the dwelling place of evil spirits.

Naming the Santa Rosas

Spanish trail-blazer Juan Bautista de Anza was probably the first of the European explorers to get a good look at the Santa Rosas—in 1774 during his historic overland trek from Mexico to Monterey. Anza and his party rounded the southern tip of the range after crossing the Colorado Desert, then paralleled the Santa Rosas to the west as they ascended Coyote Canyon. There is no record that he took more than perfunctory notice of the range. In fact, the Spaniards and their Mexican Californio successors tended to avoid the mountains of California.

The Californios apparently supplied the name for the mountains, however. "Santa Rosa" was the name given to a Mexican land grant in western Riverside County, dated 1845. This name was apparently later transferred to the mountain range. The reason is a mystery, for the Santa Rosa Mountains lie many miles south of the original land grant. Early maps of San Diego

County show the range as an extension of the San Jacintos. Not until 1901, when the U.S. Geological Survey completed its mapping of the mountains, did the name "Santa Rosa Mountains" come into general use.

Black Gold

Gold seekers were probably the first non-natives to penetrate the desert ramparts of the Santa Rosas. The earliest visitor may have been one-legged Thomas L. "Pegleg" Smith. In 1828 Smith, traveling from Yuma to Los Angeles via Warner's Ranch, left the standard route somewhere near the southern end of the Santa Rosas and sought a shortcut. The story goes that he picked up some black lumps of what he thought was native copper atop "one of three hills." In Los Angeles he showed his rocks to a friend, who suggested he have them assayed. The assayer's report: pure gold coated with "black desert varnish." Smith returned to the region where he found the rocks but was never able to locate the right spot. Ever since, an endless

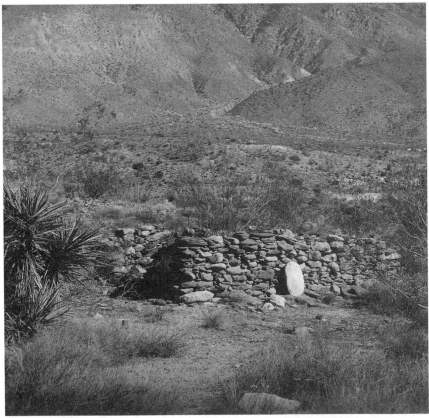

Rockhouse in Rockhouse Canyon

Charles Van Fleet

stream of prospectors have sought Pegleg Smith's fabled "black gold." The southern Santa Rosas have been "turned inside out" in a vain search that has lasted more than a century.

Pegleg's black gold may be nothing more than an elusive fable, but gold in small amounts has been brought out of the Santa Rosas. Around 1900 Nicholas Schwartz made a strike in upper Rockhouse Canyon on the southwest slope of the range. It is said that Schwartz took out $18,000 in several years work. He reportedly built and occupied one of the rock houses that gave the canyon its name. Old Nicholas Canyon, a tributary of Rockhouse Canyon, honors the old prospector today. Other prospectors have dug out minute amounts of gold from ledges in the Rockhouse Canyon area, but not enough to make their years of searching worthwhile. And there was Fig Tree John, the colorful Cahuilla who lived above the shores of the Salton Sea and died, some say, at the ripe age of 136. Old Fig Tree often made his purchases with gold dust or small nuggets, giving rise to the belief that he had a secret gold mine somewhere in the Santa Rosas. Even today, an occasional prospector sets out to find the "lost" gold mine of Fig Tree John.

The largest commercial mine in the Santa Rosas was the Garnet Queen, located at 6000 feet elevation on the northwest slope of the range. Tungsten and garnet were recovered from the Garnet Queen Mine on and off from its development in 1896 into the 1940s. The mine changed hands several time under false premises, and was a marginal success at best.

Preserving the Santa Rosas

In 1897 the entire Santa Rosa Mountains were included within the newly created San Jacinto Forest Reserve. Charlie Vandeventer, who had a cabin on what is now Vandeventer Flat, was appointed forest ranger and assigned to patrol the Santa Rosas, which, according to all accounts, he did with vigor and relish. In 1908 the old San Jacinto Reserve was cut down in size and joined to the Trabuco Reserve in the Santa Ana Mountains to form Cleveland National Forest. Only the northern end of the Santa Rosas remained as part of the Cleveland. Since 1925, this north section has been in San Bernardino National Forest. The northwestern slope, including the summit of Toro Peak, is within the Santa Rosa Indian Reservation.

Until recent years, only a handful of settlers sought homes in the desert-tempered Santa Rosas. The Vandeventer family built a cattle ranch at the northwestern foot of the range in the 1890s, and herded their stock to high mountain pastures every summer. Charley Vandeventer was for years a familiar character in these parts. A.H. Nightingale came to Pinyon Flat early in this century and built a hunting cabin at Stump Spring, high on the forested slope of Santa Rosa Mountain. Desert Steve Ragsdale, long a gas-station operator at Desert Center and later the best known dweller of the Santa Rosas, came to the mountains in 1937. He bought 560 acres of timberland atop Santa Rosa Mountain and, right on the summit, built a sturdy log cabin and a spectacular tree ladder, and posted his mountain domain with placards advising visitors, among other things, that "Decent folks are welcome; Enjoy but don't destroy." Old Desert Steve died in 1971, and his cabin burned down several years after that.

Until the 1940s the Santa Rosa Mountain–Toro Peak high country was reached only by steep trails. Since then, the road built by the Forest Service and Desert Steve Ragsdale to Santa Rosa Mountain and the later extension to Toro Peak have rendered this sylvan sky island accessible to less energetic campers and hunters. Public campgrounds have been constructed high in the forest at Santa Rosa Spring, Stump Spring and Cedar Spring.

On the lower northern slopes, subdividers are moving in. Pinyon Flat is now honeycombed with roads and new homes are springing up along the Palms-to-Pines Highway. The recently established Santa Rosa and San Jacinto Mountains National Monument aims to safeguard the pristine desert and mountain country adjacent to the new housing tracts from future development.

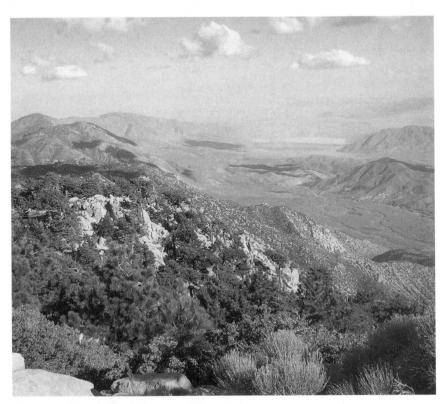

The Santa Rosa Mountains

Most of the range remains as wild as ever. South from Horsethief Creek and Toro Peak, the Santa Rosas are the lonely domain of desert bighorn sheep, coyotes and rattlesnakes. Here, often within sight of the tourist-infested Salton Sea and Anza-Borrego Desert State Park, you can wander for days, with only the wind, the soft rustle of pinyon needles, and the occasional coyote howl to keep you company.

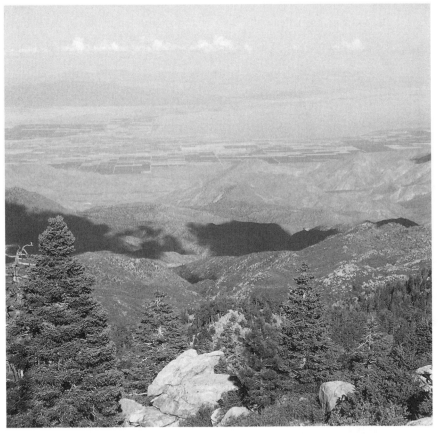

The Salton Sea from Toro Peak

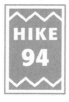

ALTA SECA BENCH

Hike Length: 8 miles round trip; 800' elevation gain
Difficulty: Moderate
Season: May–November
Topo map: *Toro Peak* (7.5')

Features

Southeast from Toro Peak, the sky island of the Santa Rosas extends 3 miles before plunging abruptly to desert canyons and foothills. This section of undisturbed high country is known to old-timers as Alta Seca Bench, although it is not so labeled on maps. Little shallow valleys filled with Jeffrey pine and live oak lie under rocky outcroppings and gentle, chaparral-spotted slopes. It is a place where you can find natural beauty and solitude, and, from its edge, gaze far out over the desert.

No maintained trails reach into the Alta Seca, and about the only visitors nowadays are occasional deer hunters during the fall. But you can find traces of the historic old Cahuilla pathway that climbed out of Horsethief Canyon, crossed the bench, and descended to Old Santa Rosa, a long-abandoned Cahuilla village near the head of Rockhouse Canyon. This trail is too ancient and overgrown to follow with certainty today. You can read about it in Charles Francis Saunders' chapter "Old Santa Rosa" in his *Southern Sierras of California;* in George Wharton James' "Up Martinez Canyon" in *Wonders of the California Desert,* and, more recently, in Nina Paul Shumway's "Burrowing in the Santa Rosas" in her *Your Desert and Mine.* These books offer delightful introductions to the Santa Rosa high country and the Native American trails that once crisscrossed it.

This cross-country trip leaves Santa Rosa Mountain Road below Toro Peak and drops to Alta Seca Bench, then crosses it to a delightful pine flat at the southeastern end. Here you can look down into Rockhouse Basin and see the route the Cahuilla took to Old Santa Rosa. (Unless you're an experienced mountaineer and are equipped for a 2-day trip, don't try to descend the old pathway.) There is no water on Alta Seca (High Dry) Bench, so tote at least two quarts of water.

Description

From Palm Desert drive up the Palms-to-Pines Highway (State Highway 74) to a junction with the Santa Rosa Mountain Road 7S02 just west of mile marker 74 RIV 77.00, marked by a large sign. Turn left (south) and proceed via the poor dirt road (high clearance recommended) up the mountainside. At 9.6 miles, you will pass the turnoff on the right to Santa Rosa's summit (on the return trip you may wish to turn off here and drive the mile up to Desert Steve Ragsdale's former mountaintop cabin and tree ladder). At 10.3

miles, you will reach a gate, which is normally locked (**GPS SB94**). Park at a wide spot in the road just below the gate where you won't block traffic.

Proceed on foot 1 mile past the locked gate, up the dirt road, staying right at the first fork, to a second fork just before the main road turns right to climb to the top of Toro Peak. Go left 0.25 mile to a dead end. From here on it's cross-country. Descend southeast 1 mile over rocky terrain spotted with pines and chaparral to Alta Seca Bench. Then follow the bench southeast 2 more miles, staying to the right (southwest) of several boulder outcroppings, to a shallow bowl filled with Jeffrey pines and some live oaks. Here, in a parklike setting, is an ideal picnic spot. To look down, climb to the rocky rim immediately south of the shallow valley. The old Native American trail dropped south down a steep ridge to Old Santa Rosa, nestled at the head of the large desert basin you see below you.

Return the same way, with an 800-foot gain at the end. Cross-country travel can be deceptive; if you're not certain of your return route, head up for the right (north) shoulder of Toro Peak, which looms high before you. Toro Peak itself is on the Santa Rosa Indian Reservation and the tribe has requested that hikers do not visit the summit.

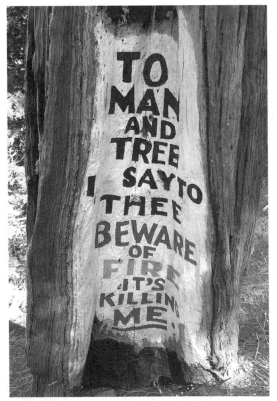

Poetry by Desert Steve

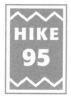

HORSETHIEF CREEK

Hike Length: 5 miles round trip; 900' elevation gain
Difficulty: Moderate
Season: November–April
Topo maps: *Toro Peak* (7.5')

Features

The northeastern end of the Santa Rosas is high desert country, ideal for winter hiking trips. Vast sloping benches and boulder-laced hills are dotted with pinyon pine, juniper, red shank, chamise, yucca, agave, and prickly pear. Shady cottonwoods grow in stream-watered canyons and around seeping springs. The snow-crowned Santa Rosa Mountain–Toro Peak massif dominates the southwestern skyline, while white-capped San Jacinto glimmers on the northern horizon.

This leisurely trip samples a small bit of this delightful high desert region. You follow the Cactus Spring Trail, an old Cahuilla pathway recently reworked by the Forest Service, from near the Palms-to-Pines Highway down into the shady gorge of Horsethief Creek. Here, amid tall cottonwoods and willows, alongside the trickling stream, you can picnic and enjoy the solitude of nature.

Horsethief Creek is wrapped in the lore of the Old West. A century ago, it is said, horsethieves used this canyon as a hideout and a place to rebrand stolen stock. Gangs of rustlers stole the horses in the San Diego region and drove them to Horsethief Creek where the animals were re-branded, then herded them to San Bernardino to sell. Before the horses could leave San Bernardino, the story goes, the bandits stole the animals back and went through the entire process in reverse.

Description

From Palm Desert drive up the Palm-to-Pines Highway (State Highway 74) to mile marker 74 RIV 80.50 at Pinyon Flat. Opposite the campground road, turn left (south) onto a paved side road (7S09, also labeled Pinyon Flats Trans Station Road). A highway sign indicates the Ribbonwood Equestrian Park and the Sawmill Trail, a new footpath leading south. Drive up 7S09 0.3 mile to the vast Sawmill Trail parking area on the left (**GPS SB95**). A sign at the east end of the lot points to the Cactus Spring Trail (5E01) and the Sawmill Trail (5E03).

Hike east from the lot. Stay right as the road turns to dirt and passes through a field of prickly pear cactus and yucca. Go 0.1 mile and stay right at another fork. Shortly after, you will see the signed Cactus Spring trailhead marker on the left. Take it; the 4WD road continuing south goes to the Sawmill Trail (see Hike 97). Follow the Cactus Spring trail east, up and down over several small north-draining gullies, and drop to Horsethief Creek, 2 miles. Here is an all-year stream shaded by magnificent cottonwoods. You can explore up or down Horsethief Creek for quite some distance.

Return the same way.

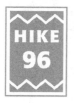

CACTUS SPRING TRAIL

HIKE 96

Hike Length: 18 miles round trip; 2400' elevation gain
Difficulty: Moderate (2 days), Strenuous (1 day)
Season: November–April
Topo maps: *Toro Peak, Martinez Mtn.* (all 7.5')

Features

This trip follows the Cactus Spring Trail from near the Palms-to-Pines Highway down across Horsethief Creek, then up over miles of rolling plateau country covered by an elfin forest of pinyon and juniper, to Agua Alta Spring. Agua Alta (High Water) Spring, creased into the south slope of Martinez Mountain, flows sparingly over green slime among cat's-claw bushes and bunch grass—not much to look at, but a heaven-sent source of water for the bighorn sheep that roam this region. Keep a sharp lookout; you may spot some of these noble animals climbing the rocky slopes of Martinez Mountain or coming down for water.

Description

From Palm Desert drive up the Palm-to-Pines Highway (State Highway 74) to mile marker 74 RIV 80.50 at Pinyon Flat. Opposite the campground road, turn left (south) onto a paved side road (7S09, also labeled Pinyon Flats Trans Station Road). A highway sign indicates the Ribbonwood Equestrian Park and the Sawmill Trail, a new footpath leading south. Drive up 7S09 0.3 mile to the vast Sawmill Trail parking area on the left (**GPS SB95**). A sign at the east end of the lot points to the Cactus Spring Trail (5E01) and the Sawmill Trail (5E03).

Hike east from the lot. Stay right as the road turns to dirt and passes through a field of prickly pear cactus and yucca. Go 0.1 mile and stay right at another fork. Shortly after, you will see the signed Cactus Spring Trailhead marker on the left. Take it; the 4WD road continuing south goes to the Sawmill Trail (see Hike 97). You follow the Cactus Spring Trail east, up and down over several small north-draining gullies, and drop to Horsethief Creek, 2 miles. Here is an all-year stream shaded by magnificent cottonwoods.

The trail crosses the creek, climbs steeply east out of the canyon, follows a dry wash, and climbs through sloping, pinyon-dotted terrain to Cactus Spring, 2 miles from Horsethief Creek. The spring, 25 yards north of the trail, is often dry. Your trail continues east, turns left up a broad, sandy wash, curves southeast up a tributary wash, and climbs toward the ridge south of Martinez Mountain. You cross the ridge well above its low point and descend into a series of dry washes leading southeast. The path climbs and descends through rough pinyon-and-juniper terrain to Agua Alta Spring, marked by a wooden sign, 6 miles from Horsethief Creek. The trickling spring is about 100 yards up the draw to your left. Enough water is almost always available here for drinking and cooking. About 0.5 mile farther on is Pinyon Alta Flat and its campsites.

Return the same way. An option is to scramble north up the long slope to the rocky summit block of Martinez Mountain, 5 miles round trip from Agua Alta Spring. A very interesting option, with a car shuttle, is to descend southeastward, following the Indian Trail, into Martinez Canyon, then follow the broad canyon around to the northeast all the way out to State Highway 86. A variation is to descend east from Pinyon Alta Flat into Agua Alta Canyon, then follow this canyon to its junction with Martinez Canyon and on out to the highway. Old trails descend both of these desert canyons. For these last two options, you will need the *Clark Lake NE* and *Valerie* (7.5′) quadrangle maps and good cross-country navigation skills. The Martinez Canyon jeep trail used to access the eastern end of Martinez Canyon from 66th Ave. and Jackson, but the northern end is now lost in a maze of new ranch development.

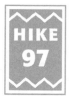

SAWMILL TRAIL

HIKE 97

Hike Length: 8 miles one way; 3700' elevation gain
Difficulty: Strenuous
Season: March–May, October–November
Topo maps: *Toro Peak* (7.5')

Features

The Sawmill Trail ascends the north face of the Santa Rosa Mountains. It provides excellent views of the northern Santa Rosas, San Jacinto, and the desert from Palm Springs southward. It starts in the desert and ends in the high mountains, so hike this trail in the spring or fall when the temperatures are cool enough at the trailhead but the Santa Rosa Mountain Road is clear of snow.

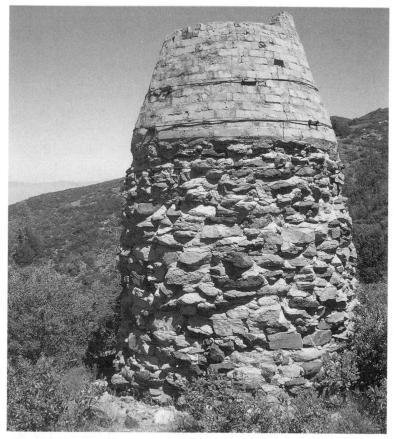

Kiln on Sawmill Trail

Description

From Palm Desert drive up the Palm-to-Pines Highway (State Highway 74) to mile marker 74 RIV 80.50 at Pinyon Flat. Opposite the campground road, turn left (south) onto a paved side road (7S09, also labeled Pinyon Flats Trans Station Road). A highway sign indicates the Ribbonwood Equestrian Park and the Sawmill Trail, a new footpath leading south. Drive up 7S09 0.3 mile to the vast Sawmill Trail parking area on the left (**GPS SB95**). A sign at the east end of the lot points to the Cactus Spring Trail (5E01) and the Sawmill Trail (5E03). You may wish to leave a second vehicle (or mountain bike) 8.7 miles up the Santa Rosa Mountain Road at the signed 5E03 trail near a bend in the road and a small gate (**GPS SB97B**).

From the Cactus Spring parking area, walk east, staying right as the road turns to dirt. Pass through a field of prickly pear cactus and yucca. After 0.1 mile, stay right at another fork. Shortly afterward, you will see the Cactus Spring Trailhead marker 5E01 to the left (see Hike 95). Stay right on the Sawmill Road 7S01 and hike north as it switchbacks up the face of the slope. Watch the flora transition as you climb from desert to mountain.

At 5.6 miles, reach a clearing at 6250' with an old stone charcoal kiln (**GPS SB97A**). From here, the 4WD road deteriorates into a trail that continues westward. After about half a mile, it forks. Stay left on the newly constructed connector trail, which climbs southwestward another 2 miles to the Santa Rosa Mountain Road.

Many variations are possible on this hike. To avoid a car shuttle, retrace your steps from the kiln or from the mountain road. With a 4WD vehicle, it is possible to drive up the Sawmill Road to the kiln and greatly shorten the hike. However, portions of the road are treacherous and the Forest Service hopes to eventually close the road to motorized vehicles. From the top of the connector trail, it is also possible to climb all the way to Santa Rosa Mountain.

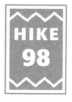

RABBIT PEAK FROM COACHELLA VALLEY

HIKE 98

Hike Length: 16 miles round trip; 6700' elevation gain
Difficulty: Very Strenuous
Season: October–April
Topo map: *Rabbit Peak* (7.5'),
Anza-Borrego Desert Region (Earthwalk)

Features

Rising high over the southern end of the Santa Rosas, overlooking Anza-Borrego Desert State Park on one side and the Salton Sea on the other, is the 6640-foot hogback of Rabbit Peak. Pinyon, juniper, and mountain mahogany cover the higher parts of this desert mountain, while the arid lower slopes are spotted with ocotillo, agave, yucca, prickly pear, and other Lower Sonoran types of plants.

Rabbit Peak is a long, tough climb. No trails reach above its desert foothills; to reach its summit you must scramble up steep, cactus-infested slopes and traverse to the north end of its long hogback. Yet it seems to hold a strange attraction to climbers, and there are those who return to this dry, unspectacular mountain time and again. In fact, it seems somehow to inspire the grandest and most touching literary artistry—exemplified in the epic poem "Wild Rabbit" written by Los Angeles Sierra Clubber Chester Versteeg, placed in the summit register in 1948:

> You sneak up on him, mile by mile,
> Foot by foot, bit by bit.
> Four jaws are grim, there's no smile;
> Then a final lunge and you've captured it—
>
> THE RABBIT!

> For seasoning use sage or wild pea,
> And, if you want to pep it up a bit,
> Dip the meat yonder in the Salton Sea.
> Yum yum, boys and girls, this is it—
>
> THE WILD RABBIT!

> Telescope, White Mountain, Boundary or New York Butte,[1]
> You bet, we like 'em all a bit.
> But today—no steak tough as a climber's boot;
> Today, tender and sweet, this is it —
>
> WILD RABBIT!

---

1 Other popular desert peaks.

In 1950, a Sierra Club group led by Jerry Zagorites added the following verse after climbing through clouds and cold rain:

And for flavor add snow and fog,
Even worse than Los Angeles smog.
When it is so cold the fire freezes,
And snow and sleet come on icy breezes—
                                    FROZEN WILD RABBIT!

The latest stanza is a lament by Parker Severson of Los Angeles, written in 1964:

Alas, what prompts we mortals so vain,
To pursue this mighty sore-muscle game.
Plodding with sweat and tears through storm and rain,
To crown these noble summits with our name?

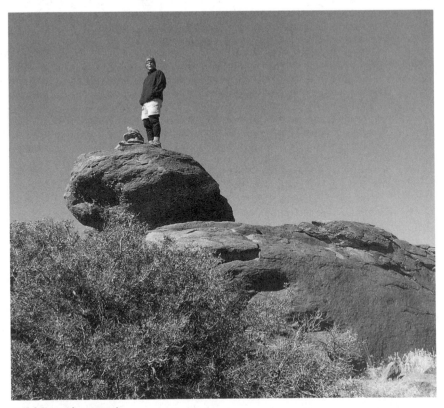

Rabbit Peak summit

Rabbit Peak can be climbed from almost any direction, a tough haul any way you do it. This trip starts from the Salton Sea side and utilizes an old prospectors' trail to gain the lower slopes. See Hike 99 for the classic but longer southern approach over Villager Peak. Take along a pen or pencil, and add your own stanza to the inspired poetry that this desert mountain seems to generate.

There is *no water* en route; take a plentiful supply. (There is a spring in Sheep Canyon which usually flows into April or May.)

Description

From Indio, drive south on State Highway 86S to the 74th Avenue junction. Make a right, then an immediate left onto Fillmore Ave. Drive south on Fillmore Avenue to its end at a gate and orchard, 2.2 miles. Park here (at **GPS SB98**). Familiarize yourself with the landmarks; you may be returning by headlamp.

Walk south over the levee and down into the wash below it. Turn right and proceed west along the wash (quite sandy in places) to where a road crosses it, 0.5 mile. Turn left (south) on the road and go about 100 yards, passing a lemon grove on your right, to a poor jeep road. Follow this road southwest about a half mile to the beginning of a well-ducked trail that leads across the open desert toward the mountains. (The trail is indistinct in places, so look for the ducks.) Your route climbs steadily southwest to the ridge between Alamo and Barton canyons, 3.5 miles. You now follow a ducked climbers' path to the left, up to the ridgetop, across a saddle, and on up to a broad, undulating bench just below the steep ridge leading up to Rabbit's hogback, 6 miles and 3300-foot gain from the start. This is where most parties camp, but it is waterless.

Beyond, it is a steep, trailless climb. Climb up the ridge around several big rock outcrops, to the top of the sloping hogback that is Rabbit Peak. You follow ducks most of the way. The register is in the summit rocks at the far (northwest) end of the plateau.

Return the same way.

VILLAGER AND RABBIT PEAKS

HIKE
99

Hike Length:	21 miles round trip; 7900' elevation gain
Difficulty:	Very Strenuous
Season:	October–April
Topo maps:	*Fonts Point, Rabbit Peak* (both 7.5'), *Anza-Borrego Desert Region* (Earthwalk)

Features

This ultimate Wild Rabbit experience ascends the long south ridge from the Anza-Borrego Desert, passing over Villager Peak en route. It is one of the testpieces for serious Southern California day hikers. This extremely strenuous hike features a remarkable variety of cactus and yucca. It is best done in late fall or early spring when the temperatures are cool. At this time of year, the hike typically begins before dawn and ends after dark, so a headlamp is essential. Fortunately, route finding is reasonably easy because the hike follows the top of the ridge. A full moon aids walking and makes the trip even more enjoyable.

The hike is completely dry. Bring at least six quarts of water, more for a warm day. Because of the plethora of spiky vegetation, long pants are advisable. The trip can be done as an overnight backpack, camping on top of Villager Peak, if you are willing to haul an enormous quantity of water.

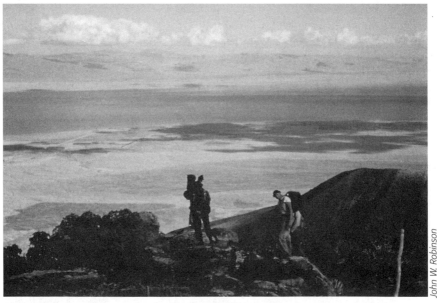

John W. Robinson

The Salton Sea, seen from the flank of Rabbit Peak

Description

From Interstate 10, turn south in Indio on Highway 86S toward El Centro and proceed for 35.5 miles to the S22 Borrego-Salton Seaway. Turn right and drive 14.8 miles to a parking area on the right at the intersection of the Thimble Trail and Truckhaven Trail dirt roads. This is just past the 32 mile marker and adjacent to call box S22-319; it is 13.1 miles east of Borrego Springs.

From the parking area, identify the ridge leading north on the left side of Rattlesnake Canyon. Wander through a maze of small washes for 1.2 miles, staying right of a small escarpment. At the base of the ridge, identify a good use trail switchbacking up the steep slope through a spectacular cactus garden. Follow this path for 5.8 miles all the way to the 5756' summit of Villager Peak.

Villager Peak is a strenuous hike in itself. If you are tired or low on water, Villager Peak is a good place to have lunch and turn around. If time permits, continue northward for 3.6 miles over numerous wearisome bumps to the 6623' summit of Rabbit Peak. The ridge involves 2000' of ascent and 1100' of descent that must be regained on the return journey.

Retrace your steps on the descent. At the 4400' point below Villager, the ridge forks. Stay to the right. The left ridge drops into complicated terrain in Rattlesnake Canyon. Once back to the desert floor, proceed south to SR22. There are numerous ducks in the desert, but none are particularly useful at night. You may occasionally see headlights on the road; head for the closest point where the lights pass by you.

OLD SANTA ROSA

Hike Length: 14 miles round trip; 2200' elevation gain
Difficulty: Moderate (2 days), Strenuous (1 day)
Season: November–April
Topo maps: *Clark Lake, Clark Lake NE, Collins Valley* (all 7.5'), *Anza-Borrego Desert Region* (Earthwalk)

Features

Charles Francis Saunders, writing in 1923, called Rockhouse Canyon "as wild a region, perhaps, as the Southern California mountains afford, scantily watered, uninhabited and unvisited except by an occasional wandering enthusiast like ourselves or a cowman in search of his strayed stock." Saunders' description holds true today. Only an occasional visitor makes the lonely trip up this narrow desert canyon to the hidden alluvial plain immediately above its head, nestled under the brooding shoulder of the Santa Rosa massif.

Years ago, this naked sloping plain above Rockhouse Canyon was the home of Mountain Cahuillas. Their village, at the northwest edge of the plain, was Old Santa Rosa. They gathered mescal from agave plants, acorns from oaks, and pinyon nuts from pines, and took water from the seeping springs below the mountainside. Although the Cahuillas have long departed and nothing remains of Old Santa Rosa, signs of their former presence are numerous. Potsherds, ollas, and other artifacts can be seen by the diligent searcher. The crumbling walls of rock houses near Cottonwood Spring (dry), however, date from a later era when Nicholas Schwarz and other prospectors combed the region for mineral wealth. From these remains Rockhouse Canyon received its name.

This wintertime trip ascends the narrow confines of Rockhouse Canyon to the lonely plain at the foot of the Santa Rosas. Chances are you will have this forgotten corner of the Santa Rosas to yourself. The only sure water is in Nicholias Canyon, just above the northwest corner of the sloping plain. You will probably need a 4-wheel drive vehicle to reach within 2 miles of Hidden Spring; the road is very poor.

Description

From Borrego Springs, follow San Diego County Road S22 east, then north, then east again to the Pegleg Smith Monument, 9.5 miles. Continue east 0.5 mile farther to an unmarked dirt road branching left (northeast) toward Clark Dry Lake. (You can also reach this junction from State Highway 86 by turning west at Salton City on the Borrego-Salton Seaway and following the latter 22 miles.) At 1.5 miles north on the before-mentioned dirt road there is another junction; go left (northwest), around the west edge of Clark Dry Lake and the strange protruding antennae of the University of Maryland Radio Telescope. In 8 miles (from S22) your road enters a rocky wash; those with low-slung vehicles may wish to park here. Continue up the wash, on rocks and soft sand, 1.5 miles farther, then turn sharp right, out of the wash, where a sign reads ROCKHOUSE CANYON. Your "road" rounds a low ridge and enters the lower reaches of Rockhouse Canyon—the absolute limit for standard cars. Jeep tracks continue another mile up-canyon until they too become impassable for any type of vehicle. Continue up the canyon on foot to Hidden Spring, marked by a wooden sign (12.5 miles from S22). Water is seldom available here.

Proceed northeast into the narrows of Rockhouse Canyon. After 3 miles, you round a bend to the north and reach the southern end of the broad, sloping plain, covered with xerophytic shrubs. Follow the dry creekbed 1 mile northwest to the remains of rock houses on your right, and 0.25 mile farther to small Cottonwood Spring. The spring is now completely dry; except for one tough cottonwood, the trees are dead. To visit the ruins of Old Santa Rosa, continue 2.5 miles to the valley's north edge, close under the abrupt wall of the Santa Rosa Mountains. The village site and its artifacts are protected by Antiquities Act of 1906. There are a few seeps at the foot of the mountain wall, but your only sure water is in Nicholias Canyon, a mile northwest.

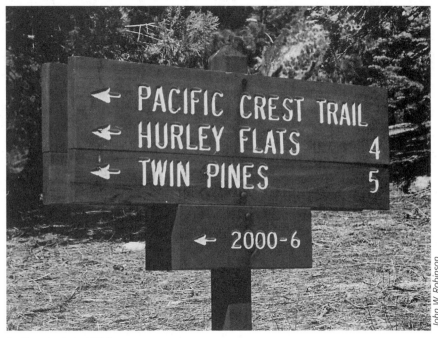

In San Jacinto Wilderness

Contacts

Information on the San Bernardino National Forest is available through the Forest Service web page www.fs.fed.us/r5/sanbernardino/contact or by contacting ranger stations directly.

San Gorgonio Wilderness:
Mill Creek Ranger Station
Highway 38 and Bryant in Mentone
34701 Mill Creek Road
Mentone, CA 92359
(909) 382-2881
8:00 A.M.–4:30 P.M. seven days a week except Thanksgiving, Christmas, New Years Day
Wilderness Permits:
www.fs.fed.us/r5/sanbernardino/documents/sgw_wilderness_permit_appl.pdf

San Jacinto Wilderness:
Idyllwild Ranger Station
Corner of Highway 243 and Pine Crest in Idyllwild
54270 Pinecrest
PO Box 518
Idyllwild, CA 92349
(909) 382-2921
8:30 A.M.–4:30 P.M. seven days a week, and most holidays

Mt. San Jacinto State Wilderness:
Mt. San Jacinto State Park Headquarters
P.O. Box 308
25905 Highway 243
Idyllwild, CA 92349
(909) 659-2607
dawn to dusk seven days a week
Wilderness Permits: www.sanjac.statepark.org/permit.html

Santa Rosa & San Jacinto Mountains National Monument
Visitor Center
Highway 74 4 miles south of Palm Desert
51-500 Highway 74
Palm Desert, CA 92260
(760) 862-9984
9:00 A.M.–4:00 P.M. seven days a week except Christmas, New Years Day

More information on the Santa Rosas is available from the Idyllwild Ranger Station for the mountain regions and from the Bureau of Land Management for the desert regions.

Bureau of Land Management (BLM)
Palm Springs South Coast Field Office
PO Box 581260
690 W. Garnet Ave.
N. Palm Springs, CA 92258-1260
(760) 251-4800

Big Bear Area
Big Bear Discovery Center
Highway 38 between Fawnskin and Stanfield Cutoff
(909) 866-3437
8:00 A.M.–6:00 P.M. Memorial Day through Labor Day
8:00 A.M.–4:30 P.M. off peak season
Open seven days a week

Lake Arrowhead Area
Skyforest Ranger Station
Highway 18 between Highway 173 and Arrowhead Villas Road
28104 Highway 18
PO Box 350
Skyforest, CA 92385
(909) 382-2782
8:30 A.M.–4:30 P.M. Monday–Saturday

Pacific Crest Trail

The Pacific Crest Trail, the most ambitious footpath in the United States, traverses the crest of the Pacific states for 2,650 miles from Mexico to Canada. The proposal to carve this wilderness path from border to border was conceived by a single individual in 1932—Clinton C. Clarke of Pasadena. He urged the Forest Service and National Park System to knit together and extend the threads of high-country footpaths already existing, such as the Oregon Skyline Trail and California's John Muir Trail. Clarke achieved partial success before his death in 1957; he prevailed upon the Forest Service to call the footpaths in Oregon and Washington by the collective name "Pacific Crest Trail System." But not until 1968, when Congress, responding to pressure from outdoorsmen, created the PCT as a national scenic trail, did active work begin to join together a border-to-border system.

The Pacific Crest Trail crosses the length of San Bernardino National Forest. The route, from south to north, goes as follows: From Anza Valley up and along the crest of Thomas Mountain, down Thomas Mountain Road to State Highway 74, north from the east end of Lake Hemet through May Valley to the South Ridge of Tahquitz Peak, over Tahquitz Peak and down to Saddle Junction, up past Wellman Cienega to San Jacinto Peak, down the Deer Springs Trail to the Fuller Ridge Trail, northwest on the latter to Black Mountain Road, down the north slope to Hurley Flat and on to San Gorgonio Pass. East to Whitewater Road, north up the Whitewater River, across the ridge to Mission Creek, up the North Fork of the latter to Heart Bar Creek, up Coon Creek and across Onyx Summit, northwest down to Big Bear City, up Van Dusen Canyon to Holcomb Valley, west to Big Pine Flat, down Holcomb Creek to Deep Creek, west north of Lake Arrowhead to Grass Valley Creek, west down the East Fork of the Mojave River to Summit Valley, west to Cajon Pass and up Lone Pine Canyon into the San Gabriels.

For more information on the Pacific Crest Trail, see *Pacific Crest Trail: Southern California*, by Schaffer, Winnett, Schifrin, and Jenkins, published by Wilderness Press.

GPS Waypoints

Global Positioning Satellite (**GPS**) coordinates for trailheads and certain other points are given in the table below. They typically have an error of less than 50 feet, but larger errors may exist. Remember that a GPS is never a substitute for good navigation skills, a map and compass, and common sense.

Reaching the start is the most difficult part of some of these trips. The author used a car-mounted Garmin StreetPilot 2610 to help locate trailheads. It contains the CityNavigator database, which includes a nearly accurate representation of almost all of the dirt roads in this book.

Waypoint	Position	Elevation	Description
SB01A	N34 18.734 W117 26.274	13927 ft	Cleghorn Trailhead
SB01B	N34 17.649 W117 24.853	5250 ft	Cleghorn Upper Trailhead
SB01C	N34 17.966 W117 27.411	2998 ft	Cleghorn Lower Trailhead
SB02	N34 16.237 W117 24.235	4983 ft	Cajon Trailhead
SB03	N34 15.426 W117 18.350	4402 ft	Seeley Creek Trailhead
SB04	N34 13.462 W117 17.978	3635 ft	Marshall Peak Trailhead
SB04A	N34 12.615 W117 18.156	4015 ft	Marshall Peak
SB05	N34 13.379 W117 16.111	4909 ft	Arrowhead Peak Trailhead
SB06	N34 21.833 W117 09.706	4519 ft	Bowen Ranch
SB07	N34 17.248 W117 12.856	4907 ft	Rock Camp Parking
SB08	N34 17.782 W117 12.678	4767 ft	Pinnacles Trailhead
SB09	N34 16.021 W117 09.771	5353 ft	Little Bear Creek Trailhead
SB09A	N34 16.168 W117 08.296	4701 ft	Little Bear Creek Trailhead 2
SB10	N34 16.282 W117 08.166	4722 ft	Deep Creek Trailhead
SB12	N34 14.025 W117 09.642	6050 ft	Heaps Peak Parking
SB13	N34 15.679 W117 06.108	5747 ft	Deep Creek Trailhead
SB14A	N34 16.618 W117 04.563	5203 ft	Holcomb Crossing Trail Camp
SB14B	N34 15.888 W117 05.408	5802 ft	Crab Flats ATV Trailhead
SB15	N34 20.070 W117 04.142	5634 ft	Coxey Creek Trailhead
SB16	N34 19.354 W117 03.505	5927 ft	Hawes Ranch Trailhead

Waypoint	Position	Elevation	Description
SB19	N34 12.141 W117 05.199	6039 ft	Exploration Trailhead
SB19A	N34 12.373 W117 02.624	7300 ft	Exploration Trailhead 2
SB20	N34 13.491 W117 02.477	6726 ft	Little Green Valley Trailhead
SB20A	N34 14.587 W117 04.139	7008 ft	Little Green Valley Trailhead 2
SB21	N34 13.473 W117 01.460	6938 ft	Camp Creek Trailhead
SB22	N34 15.781 W116 56.885	6784 ft	Grays Peak Trailhead
SB23	N34 17.021 W116 55.034	7486 ft	Delamar Mountain Trailhead
SB24	N34 15.844 W116 54.653	6873 ft	Bertha Peak Trailhead
SB24A	N34 16.981 W116 53.962	8201 ft	Bertha Peak
SB25	N34 18.179 W116 49.764	7262 ft	Gold Mountain Trailhead
SB25A	N34 18.135 W116 49.386	6910 ft	Gold Mountain Trailhead 2
SB26	N34 19.669 W116 48.954	5800 ft	Silver Peak 4WD Trailhead
SB26A	N34 19.319 W116 49.094	5851 ft	Silver Peak 2WD Trailhead
SB26B	N34 20.259 W116 48.627	6756 ft	Silver Peak
SB27A	N34 16.490 W116 44.776	6044 ft	Champion Joshua Tree 2WD Trailhead
SB27B	N34 16.485 W116 44.278	6066 ft	Champion Joshua Tree 4WD Trailhead
SB28	N34 14.263 W116 57.689	6872 ft	Castle Rock Trailhead
SB29	N34 12.922 W116 58.440	7592 ft	Lodgepole Pine Trailhead
SB31	N34 14.167 W116 55.646	6875 ft	Pineknot Trailhead
SB32	N34 13.126 W116 48.370	7520 ft	Sugarloaf Trailhead
SB33	N34 12.333 W116 45.908	8652 ft	Sugarloaf Trailhead 2
SB33A	N34 10.579 W116 45.190	7837 ft	Wildhorse Meadows Turnoff
SB34	N34 09.772 W116 47.317	6791 ft	Wildhorse Trailhead
SB34A	N34 11.357 W116 47.232	7810 ft	Wildhorse Trail Camp
SB34B	N34 10.023 W116 48.774	6495 ft	Wildhorse Creek Trailhead
SB35	N34 10.241 W116 49.792	6285 ft	Santa Ana River Trailhead
SB36	N34 08.855 W116 47.395	7424 ft	Aspen Grove Trailhead
SB37	N34 07.471 W116 46.028	8136 ft	Fish Creek Trailhead
SB38	N34 09.863 W116 54.732	6759 ft	Ponderosa Trailhead
SB39	N34 10.971 W116 59.195	4994 ft	Seven Pines Trailhead
SB40	N34 09.694 W116 52.356	6759 ft	South Fork Trailhead
SB43A	N34 05.954 W116 49.495	11502 ft	San Gorgonio Mountain
SB43B	N34 07.096 W116 51.624	10000 ft	Dollar Lake Saddle
SB46	N34 09.618 W116 53.976	6747 ft	Forsee Creek Trailhead
SB46A	N34 08.707 W116 55.525	7250 ft	Johns Meadow
SB47A	N34 07.686 W116 53.355	10601 ft	Forsee / San Bernardino Divide Junction
SB48	N34 08.775 W116 58.696	5843 ft	San Bernardino Peak Trailhead
SB48A	N34 07.341 W116 55.345	10649 ft	San Bernardino Peak
SB48B	N34 08.369 W116 56.318	8328 ft	Manzanita Springs Junction

Waypoint	Position	Elevation	Description
SB48C	N34 07.219 W116 55.859	10292 ft	Washington's Monument
SB49A	N34 07.482 W116 54.588	10691 ft	San Bernardino Peak East
SB49B	N34 07.479 W116 53.659	10864 ft	Anderson Peak
SB49C	N34 07.631 W116 52.931	10701 ft	Shields Peak
SB49D	N34 07.614 W116 52.394	10563 ft	Alto Diablo
SB49E	N34 06.888 W116 51.220	10806 ft	Charlton Peak
SB49F	N34 06.622 W116 51.027	10696 ft	Little Charlton Peak
SB49G	N34 06.177 W116 50.687	11205 ft	Jepson Peak
SB50	N34 05.226 W116 54.890	5543 ft	Momyer Trailhead
SB50A	N34 07.599 W116 54.403	10534 ft	Momyer / San Bernardino Divide Junction
SB53	N34 04.935 W116 53.600	6018 ft	Big Falls Trailhead
SB54	N34 04.927 W116 53.466	6008 ft	Vivian Creek Trailhead
SB54A	N34 05.184 W116 50.823	9235 ft	High Camp
SB54B	N34 06.083 W116 50.039	11266 ft	Vivian Creek / Sky High Junction
SB56	N34 05.721 W117 06.539	1875 ft	Cram Peak Trailhead
SB56A	N34 06.121 W117 01.469	3344 ft	Cram Peak Trailhead 2
SB57	N33 49.643 W116 47.725	5155 ft	Black Mountain Trailhead
SB57A	N33 49.591 W116 45.025	7323 ft	Black Mountain / Boulder Basin Junction
SB57B	N33 49.610 W116 45.383	7397 ft	Boulder Basin Campground
SB58	N33 50.341 W116 44.173	7753 ft	Fuller Ridge Trailhead
SB59	N33 47.820 W116 46.624	5515 ft	Indian Mountain Trailhead
SB60	N33 47.813 W116 44.469	5424 ft	San Jacinto River Parking
SB61	N33 48.595 W116 44.038	6270 ft	Seven Pines Trailhead
SB62	N33 47.476 W116 44.128	6237 ft	Marion Mountain Trailhead
SB63	N33 45.105 W116 45.542	5520 ft	Webster Trailhead
SB64	N33 45.180 W116 43.364	5603 ft	Deer Springs Trailhead
SB65A	N33 46.004 W116 41.395	6355 ft	Suicide Rock Climber Trailhead
SB67	N33 45.880 W116 41.143	6415 ft	Humber Park
SB74	N33 45.878 W116 41.220	6375 ft	Ernie Maxwell Trailhead
SB76	N33 44.415 W116 42.149	5701 ft	Ernie Maxwell Trailhead 2
SB77	N33 44.126 W116 41.761	6445 ft	South Ridge Trailhead
SB78	N33 41.863 W116 39.150	4947 ft	Spitler Peak Trailhead
SB80	N33 40.766 W116 36.849	5197 ft	Fobes Trailhead
SB81	N33 39.251 W116 35.373	5477 ft	Cedar Springs Trailhead
SB82	N33 37.261 W116 38.049	4493 ft	Ramona Trailhead
SB83	N33 35.783 W116 46.823	4495 ft	Cahuilla Mountain Trailhead
SB84	N33 50.232 W116 36.834	2591 ft	Tramway Parking
SB86	N33 49.432 W116 32.961	451 ft	Art Museum

Waypoint	Position	Elevation	Description
SB88	N33 45.990 W116 32.337	592 ft	Palm Canyon Toll Gate
SB91	N33 34.331 W116 30.053	4362 ft	Ribbonwood Palm Canyon Trailhead
SB93	N33 42.038 W116 22.484	369 ft	Living Desert Zoo
SB94	N33 31.726 W116 25.955	7813 ft	Alta Seca Bench Parking
SB95	N33 34.798 W116 27.021	4043 ft	Cactus Spring / Lower Sawmill Trailhead
SB97A	N33 33.010 W116 26.659	6232 ft	Middle Sawmill Trailhead
SB97B	N33 32.559 W116 27.942	7495 ft	Upper Sawmill Trailhead
SB98	N33 28.634 W116 07.795	-77 ft	Rabbit Peak Parking

Bibliography

General

Fletcher, Colin. *The Complete Walker*, Alfred A. Knopf, New York, 1968.

Leadabrand, Russ. *A Guidebook to the San Bernardino Mountains of California*, Ward Ritchie Press, Los Angeles, 1964 (out of print).

Manning, Harvey (ed.). *Mountaineering: The Freedom of the Hills*, The Mountaineers, Seattle, 1967.

Olander, Ann and Farley. *Call of the Mountains: The Beauty and Legacy of Southern California's San Jacinto, San Bernardino, and San Gabriel Mountains*, Stephens Press, Las Vegas, 2005.

Nature

Booth, Ernest S. *Mammals of Southern California*, U. of Calif. Press, Berkeley, 1968.

Dawson, E. Yale. *Cacti of California*, U. of Calif. Press, Berkeley, 1966.

DeLisle, Harold. *Common Plants of the Southern California Mountains*, Naturegraph Co., Healdsburg, 1961.

DeLisle, Harold. *Wildlife of the Southern California Mountains*, Naturegraph Co., Healdsburg, 1963.

Furtz, Francis. *The Elfin Forest*, Times-Mirror Press, Los Angeles, 1923.

Grinnell, Joseph. *Biota of the San Bernardino Mountains*, U. of Calif. Publ. in Zoology, Berkeley, 1908.

Grinnell, Joseph and H.S. Swarth. *Birds and Mammals of the San Jacinto Area*, U. of Calif. Publ. in Zoology, Berkeley, 1913.

Hall, Harvey M. *A Botanical Survey of San Jacinto Mountain*, U. of Calif. Publ. in Botany, Berkeley, 1902.

Kenline, George A. *Familiar Trees of the San Bernardino Mountains*, Grizzly Press, Big Bear Lake, 1971.

Munz, Philip. *California Mountain Wildflowers*, U. of Calif. Press, Berkeley, 1963.

Peterson, P. Victor. *Native Trees of Southern California*, U. of Calif. Press, Berkeley, 1966.

Raven, Peter H. *Native Shrubs of Southern California*, U. of Calif. Press, Berkeley, 1966.

Sudworth, George. *Forest Trees of the Pacific Slope*, Dover Publications, New York, 1967 (reprint of 1908 edition).

Vaughn, Francis E. *Geology of the San Bernardino Mountains North of San Gorgonio Pass*, U. of Calif. Publ. in Geology, Berkeley, 1922.

History

Beattie, George William & Helen Pruitt. *Heritage of the Valley: San Bernardino's First Century*, San Pasqual Press, Pasadena, 1939.

Beldon, Burr, "History in the Making." San Bernardino Sun-Telegram, various issues, 1953–1964.

Big Bear Panorama. Big Bear High School, Big Bear, 1934.

Brown, John, Jr., & James Boyd. *History of San Bernardino and Riverside Counties*, Lewis Publ. Co., Chicago, 1922.

Drake, Austin. *Big Bear Valley: Its History, Legends and Tales*, Big Bear Historical Society, Big Bear, 1970 (reprint of 1949 edition).

Holmes, Elmer W. *History of Riverside County, California*, Historic Record Co., Los Angeles, 1912.

Hughes, Tom. *History of Banning and San Gorgonio Pass*, Banning Record, Banning, (1939).

Ingersoll, Luther A. *Century Annals of San Bernardino County, 1769–1904*, Ingersoll, Los Angeles, 1904.

Jackson, Helen Hunt. *Ramona*, Little, Brown & Co., Boston, 1884.

James, George Wharton. *Through Ramona's Country*, Little, Brown & Co., Boston, 1909.

James, George Wharton. *Wonders of the Colorado Desert*, Little, Brown & Co., Boston, 1906.

James, Harry C. *The Cahuilla Indians*, Westernlore Press, Los Angeles, 1960 (reprinted 1969 by Malki Museum Press, Banning).

Johnson, Frank. *The Serrano Indians of Southern California*, Malki Museum Press, Banning, 1965.

La Fuze, Pauliena. *Saga of the San Bernardinos*, San Bernardino County Museum Association, 1971.

Maxwell, Ernest (ed.). *The Town Crier* (newspaper); Idyllwild, various issues, 1946–1971.

Patencio, Chief Francisco (told to Margaret Boynton). *Stories and Legends of the Palm Springs Indians*, Palm Springs Desert Museum, Palm Springs, 1970 (reprint of 1943 edition).

Robinson, John. *The San Bernardinos*, Big Santa Anita Historical Society, Arcadia, CA, 1989.

Robinson, John. *San Gorgonio: A Wilderness Preserved*, The San Gorgonio Volunteer Association, San Bernardino, 1991.

Robinson, John & Bruce Risher. *The San Jacinto*, Big Santa Anita Historical Society, Arcadia, CA, 1993.

Ruby, Jay W. *Aboriginal Uses of Mt. San Jacinto State Park*, U.C.L.A. Dept. of Anthropology Annual Publ., Los Angeles, 1961–62.

Saunders, Charles F. *The Southern Sierras of California*, Houghton-Mifflin Co., Boston, 1923.

Shumway, Nina Paul. *Your Desert and Mine*, Westernlore Press, Los Angeles, 1960.

Williamson, Robert S. *Report of Explorations in California for Railroad Routes*, War Dept., Washington, 1853.

Woodward, Lois Ann. *Mount San Jacinto*, W.P.A. Project, Berkeley, 1937 (typescript in Bancroft Library).

INDEX

About the Authors

John W. Robinson has explored, back-packed, and climbed throughout the mountain west, from Alaska and Canada to Mexico, for over 50 years. His first guide, *Camping and Climbing in Baja* (now out of print) set the standard for guides to the Baja California mountains. His *Trails of the Angeles*, now in its eighth edition, remains the definitive hiking guide to southern California's San Gabriel Mountains.

He has authored or co-authored a number of the original Wilderness Press quadrangle guides, covering California's three major southern ranges: the San Gabriels, the San Bernardinos, and the San Jacintos. In addition, he has published numerous articles in *Westways*, *Desert Magazine*, *The Southern California Quarterly*, *The Overland Journal*, and *Summit*.

If the mines of southern California's mountains revealed gold and other precious minerals, they cannot compare to the treasure trove of information contained in this one man. His love for these forests, peaks, and wilderness areas is apparent on every page of his many works.

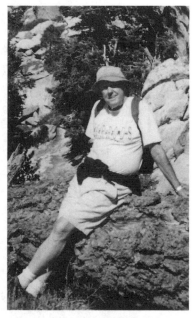

John Robinson on Fuller Ridge

David Money Harris teaches Engineering at Harvey Mudd College. When he is not in class, he can often be found hiking or climbing. He is the author of three books on integrated circuit design. He is delighted to explore the Southern California mountains while revising this book. His son, Abraham, was born during this writing project and has already helped scout five of the hikes.

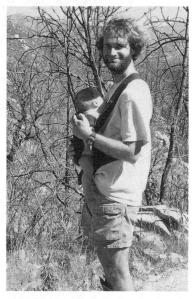

David Money Harris (& Abraham)

Also available from WILDERNESS PRESS

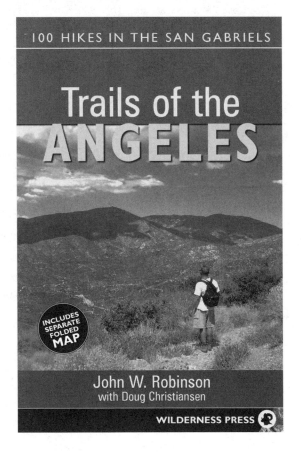

The classic guide to the San Gabriel Mountains features 100 hikes ranging from one-hour strolls to weekend backcountry trips. *Trails of the Angeles* includes trips in Angeles National Forest, as well as a few in San Bernardino National Forest, plus fascinating historical and natural-history notes and a sheet map showing all the hikes described in the book.

ISBN 0-89997-377-9

For ordering information, contact your local bookseller or
Wilderness Press, www.wildernesspress.com